LOW FODMAP GUT-BOOSTING RECIPES & 14 DAY MEAL PLAN

Making your FODMAP Life easy!

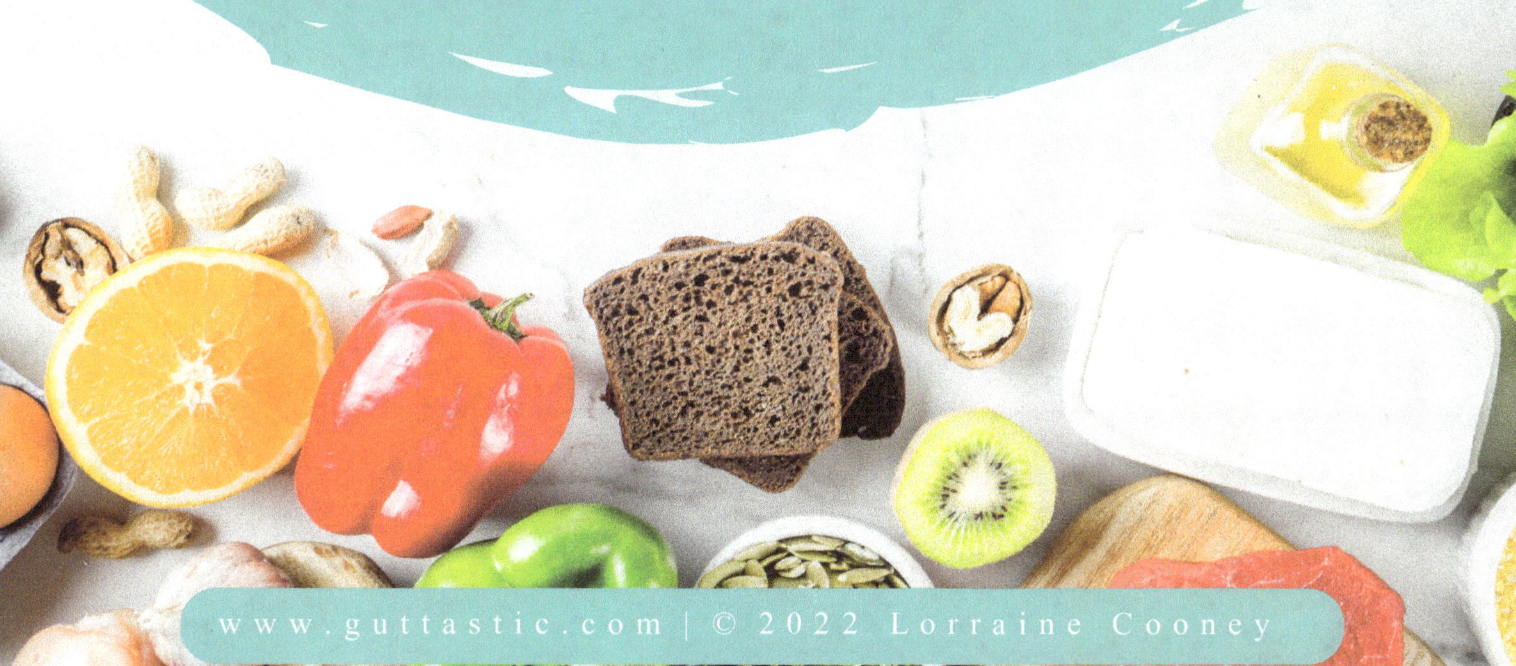

LOW FODMAP MEAL PLAN & RECIPES

Making your FODMAP Life easy!

This eBook is for information and education purposes only

You should not use the information in this eBook to diagnose any health problem or illness

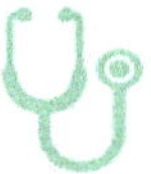

This eBook does not replace personlalised nutrition or medical advice

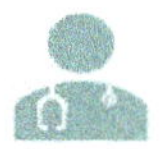

It is recommended to seek advice from your dietitian or doctor before implementing the dietary changes

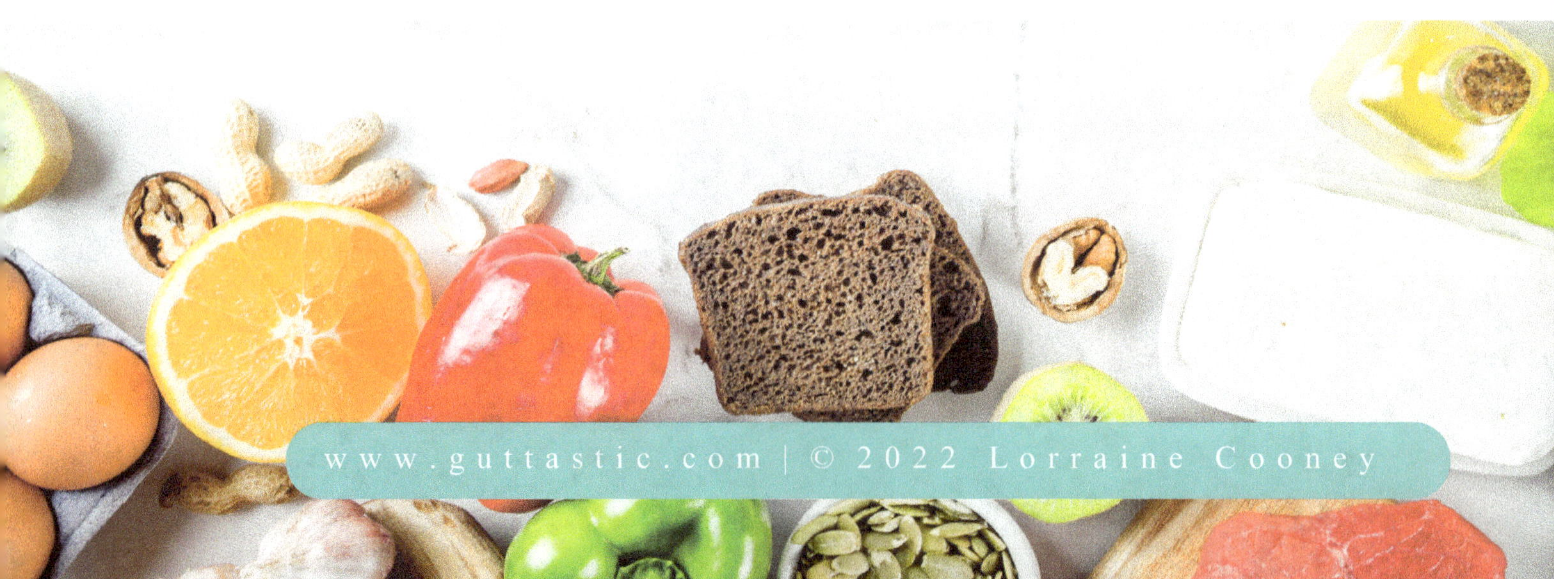

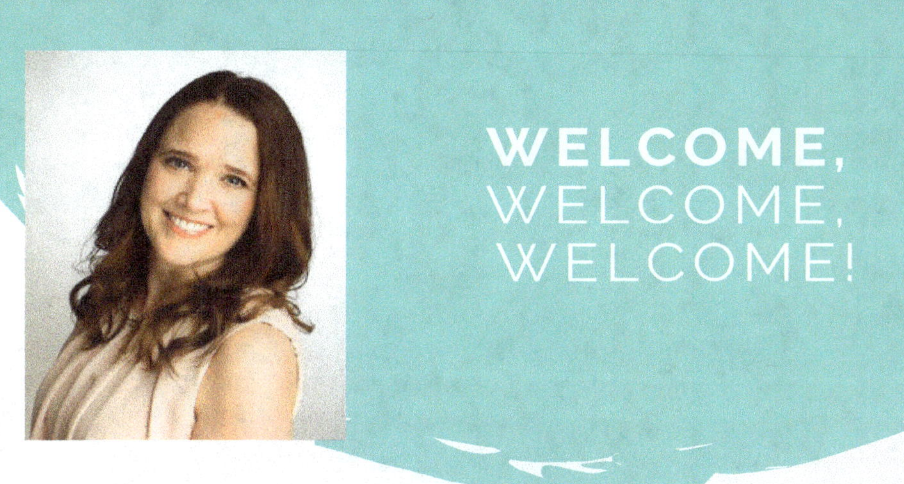

I'm Lorraine, an IBS & Gut Health dietitian with a passion for helping people dominate their digestive condition and gain control of unwanted gut symptoms, to be free to live their best life!

My passion is also my mission: To help people have agency over their digestive condition and find freedom from food-based anxiety - which can have a profound effect on one's mental wellbeing and life choices. People often need to compromise their life to accommodate gut symptoms, so my goal is to help remove any unnecessary limitations on the choices a person can make about how they want to live. .

Following a low FODMAP diet can be tricky and impact your relationship with food. Research indicates that a low FODMAP diet is best used under the supervision of a dietitian, to support the personalisation of your plan and overcome some of the potential pitfalls and risks, such as negative changes in the levels of beneficial bacteria and lack of gut loving fibre in your diet.

This eBook contains over 50 easy gut friendly low FODMAP recipes so that you go through the FOMDAP diet, keeping one eye on following the restriction and one eye on maintaining gut health! There is also space to plan your shopping list, meals and make notes.

Happy cooking!

Lorraine x

Lorraine Cooney
Founder of www.guttastic.com

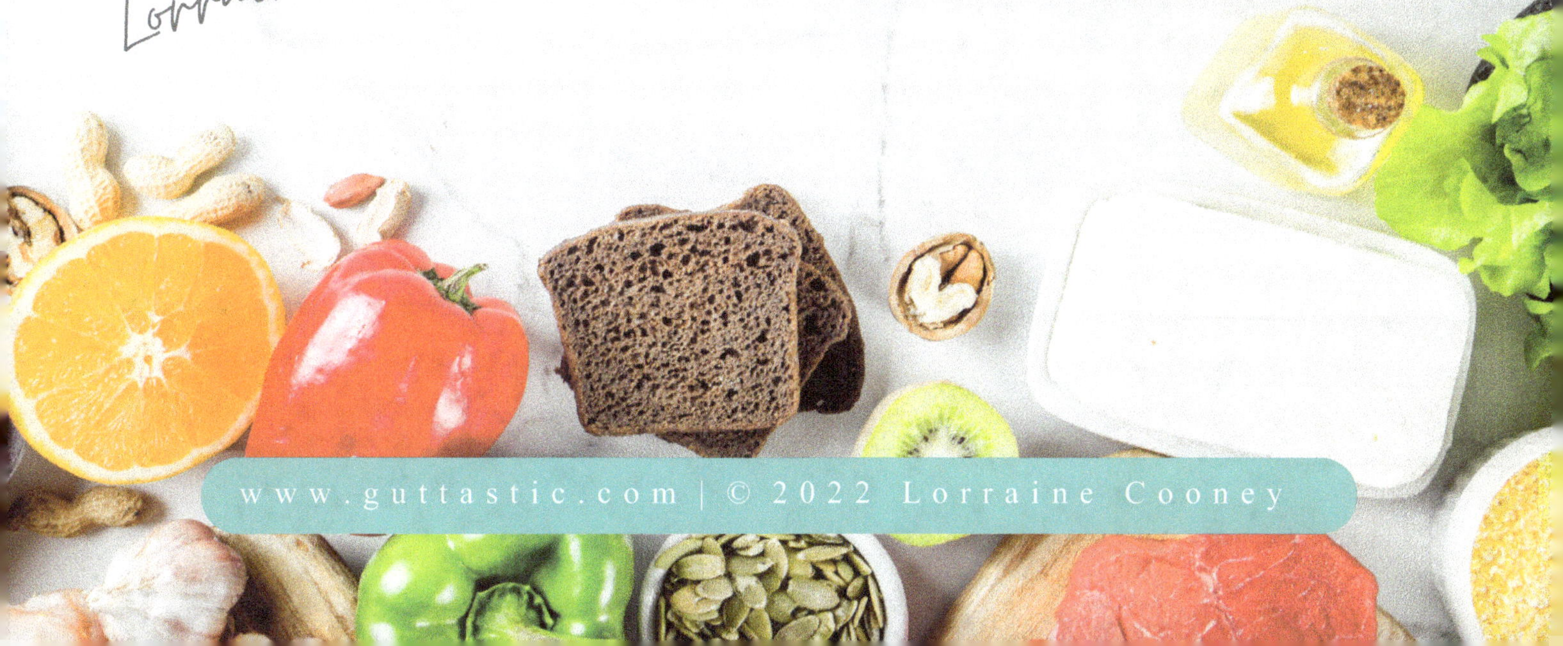

14 DAY MEAL PLAN

	Breakfast	Lunch	Dinner
Week 1			
1	Chia Seed Pudding	Minestrone Soup	Chicken Fried Rice
1	Strawberry Overnight Oats	Tuna & artichoke Salad	Spinach and Feta frittata
3	Mixed Seed Granola	Quinoa Tabbouleh	Pizza with 'Mix n Match' Toppings
4	Tofu-Feta Scramble	Veg-tastic Omelette	Spaghetti Bolognese
5	Frozen Yoghurt Breakfast Bark	Kimchi Fried Rice	Ginger and Soya Salmon
6	Raspberry Pancakes	Peanut-Tofu Buddha Bowl	Pasta with prawns
7	Fibre Power Oatmeal	Miso Roasted Veg with Lentils	Moroccan Chicken
Week 2			
8	Avo-Egg on Toast	Kimchi Pancakes	Halloumi Tray Bake
9	Buckwheat Pancakes	Chickpea Pasta salad	Coconut Fish Curry
10	Fancy French Toast	Thai Inspired Prawn Soup	Chicken and Lentil Stew
11	Flourless Banana Pancakes	Low FODMAP Falafels	Beetroot & Goats Cheese Risotto
12	A 'Live' & Kickin' Strawberry	Caprese Salad	Tasty Tofu Stir Fry
13	FODMAP Brekkie Bars	Rainbow Halloumi Wraps	Peanut Quinoa Stew
14	Egg Shakshuka	Gut Nourishing Lunch Bowls	Saag Paneer

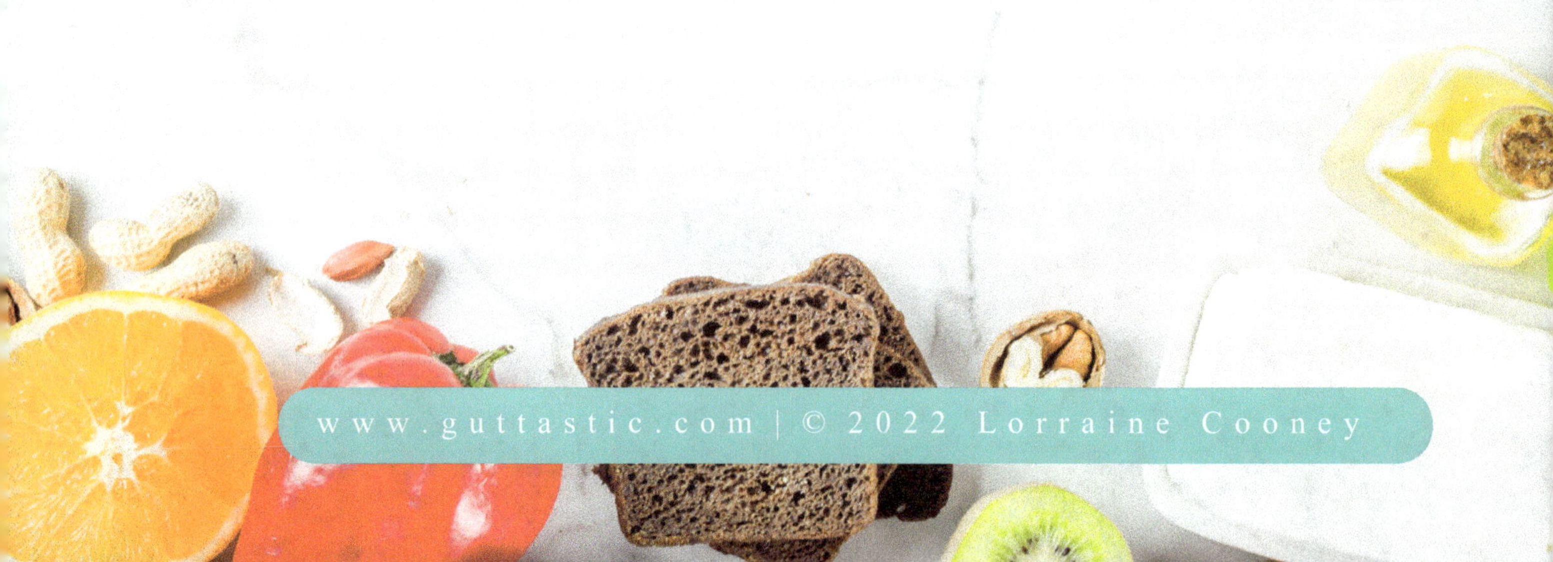

BREAKFAST

Making your FODMAP Life easy!

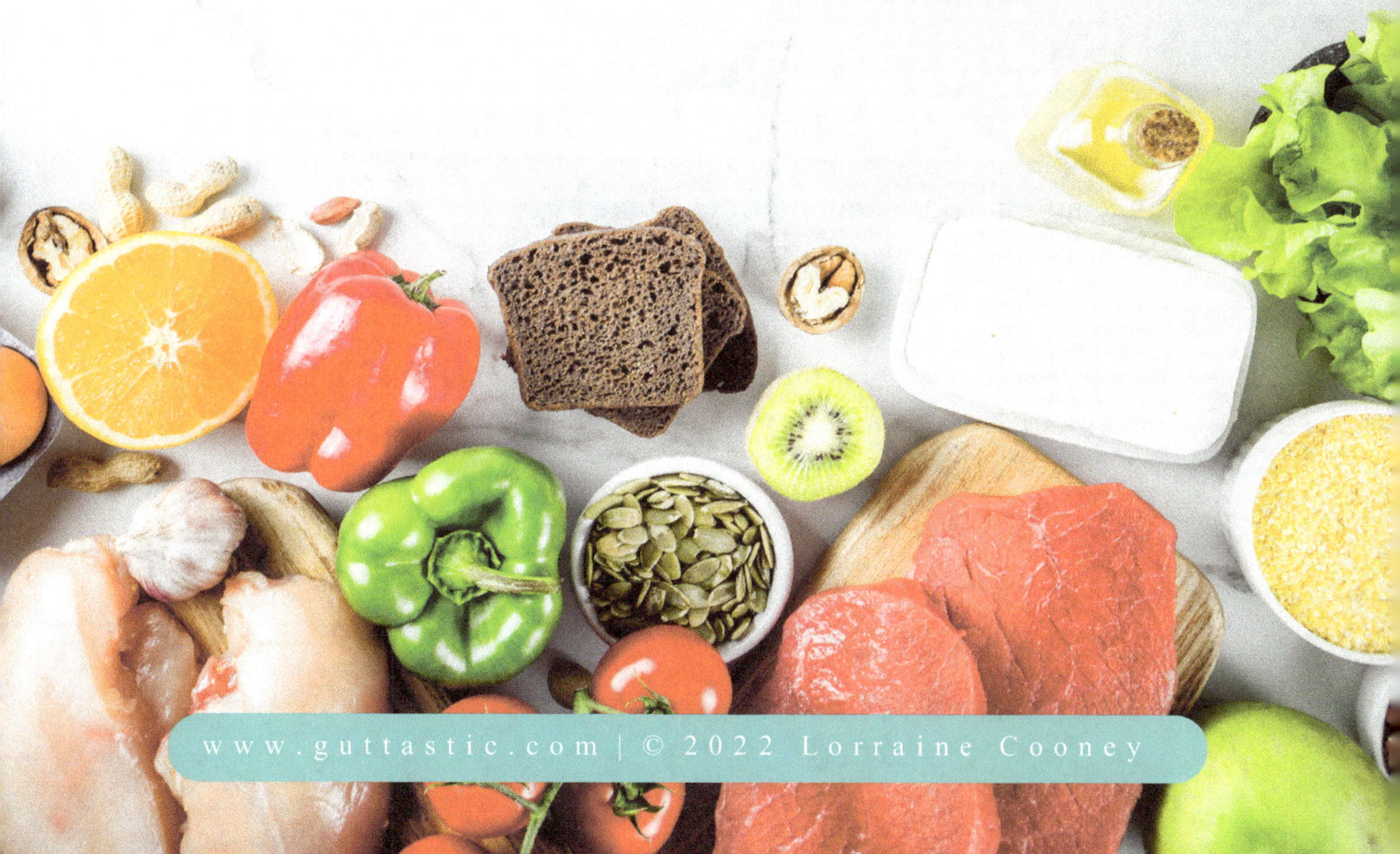

Chia Seed
Pudding
Serves 1

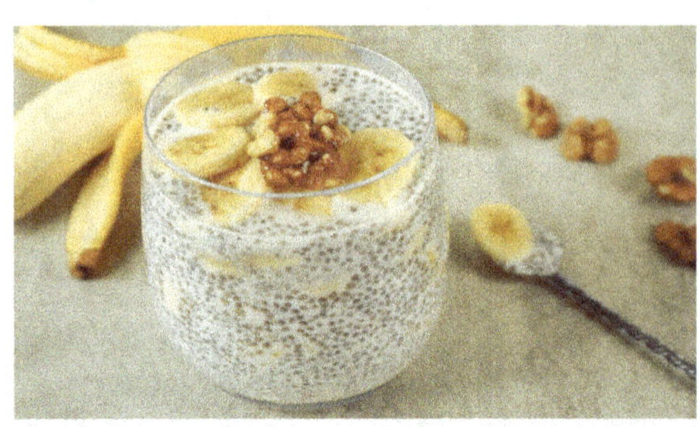

Ingredients

3 tbs chia seeds
250ml lactose free or almond milk
1 tbs maple syrup
1/4 tsp ground cinnamon
1/2 tsp almond extract

Toppings:
Unripe banana, sliced
Handful of walnuts

Directions

1. In a medium bowl or large measuring cup combine all ingredients (except toppings) and stir to combine
2. Seal the container and place in the fridge for 4 hours or longer (the longer you let it sit, the more the chia seeds will also soften and expand)
3. When ready to serve, top with banana and walnuts
4. Keeps to 3 days in the refrigerator

Strawberry Overnight Oats

Serves 1

Ingredients

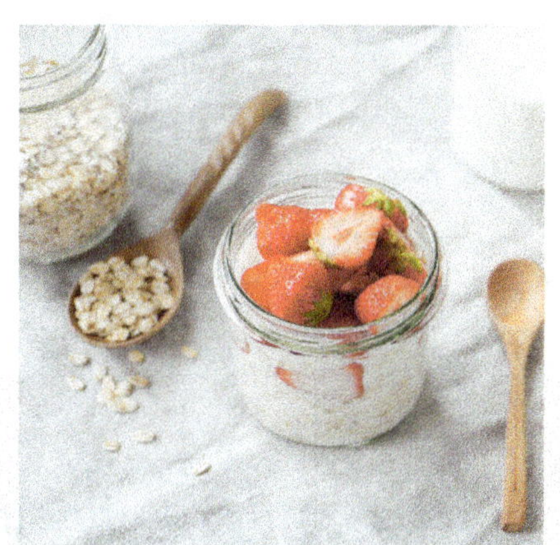

40g oats
150g pot strawberry lactose free or dairy free yoghurt
50g strawberries (fresh or frozen)
1 tbs flaxseeds seeds
1 tsp vanilla essence

Directions

1. Stir all ingredients together in a sealable jar or cover with cling film
2. Place in the fridge overnight
3. Add some extra strawberries before serving, if desired

Mixed Seed Granola

Serves 6

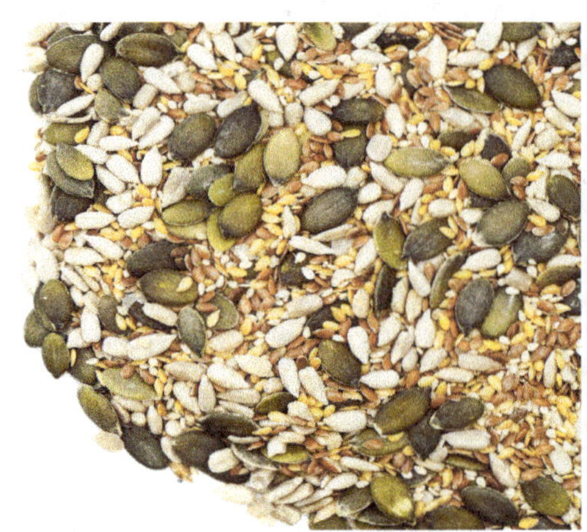

Ingredients

420g porridge oats
100g mixed seeds
50g pecans,chopped
50g desiccated coconut
45ml olive oil
45ml maple syrup
1 tsp vanilla extract
½ tsp ground cinnamon

Directions

1. Mix the oats, seeds, nuts and coconut in a large bowl.
2. Gently warm the oil and syrup together and add the vanilla essence
3. Combine the wet and dry ingredients and lay out evenly on baking tray.
4. Cook at 180°C for 20-25 minutes or until its nicely toasted.
5. Store in an airtight container for the week

Tofu-Feta Scramble

Serves 2-3

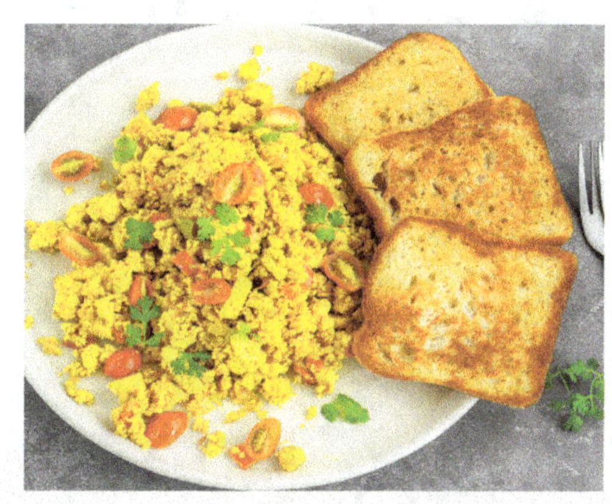

Ingredients

1 tbs extra virgin olive oil
300g extra-firm tofu, patted dry
8 cherry tomatoes, halved
2 tbs nutritional yeast
½ tsp salt
½ tsp ground cumin
½ tsp turmeric

4 spring onions, green part only
Black pepper
100g feta cheese, crumbled
Handful fresh coriander leaves

Directions

1. Add oil to a non-stick pan on medium heat.
2. Crumble in the tofu and add the tomatoes, nutritional yeast, spices, thyme and season taste
3. Cook the tofu mix in a frying pan, stirring occasionally, until heated through and getting a bit browned, about 4-5 minutes.
4. Sprinkle with chopped spring onion and feta and cook for about 30 seconds more
5. Sprinkle with coriander leaves and serve with your favourite bread

Frozen Yoghurt Breakfast Bark

Serves 4

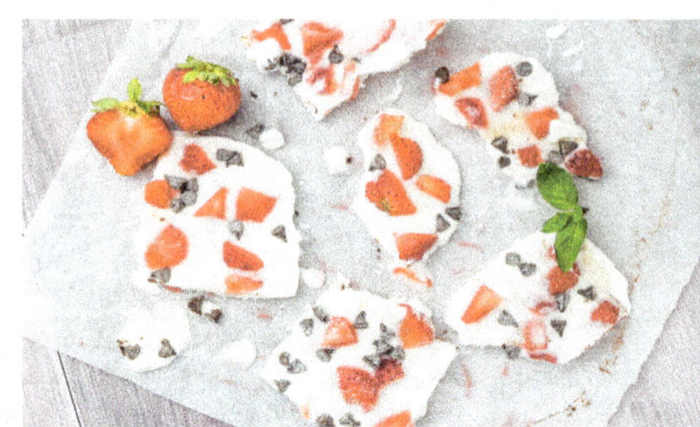

Ingredients

120g Greek yoghurt or lactose free yoghurt
½ tsp vanilla extract
¼ tsp fresh lemon juice
Handful of chopped pecans
40 chopped almonds
6 sliced strawberries
2 tbs dried cranberries

Directions

1. Line a baking sheet with baking paper.
2. In a large mixing bowl combine yogurt, vanilla extract, lemon juice and whisk until thoroughly combined.
3. Transfer yogurt mixture to the prepared baking sheet and spread it around to an even thickness.
4. Top with berries and nuts
5. Freeze for 2 to 3 hours, or until firm.
6. Cut into pieces and serve.
7. Keep in the freezer

Raspberry Pancakes

Serves 2-3

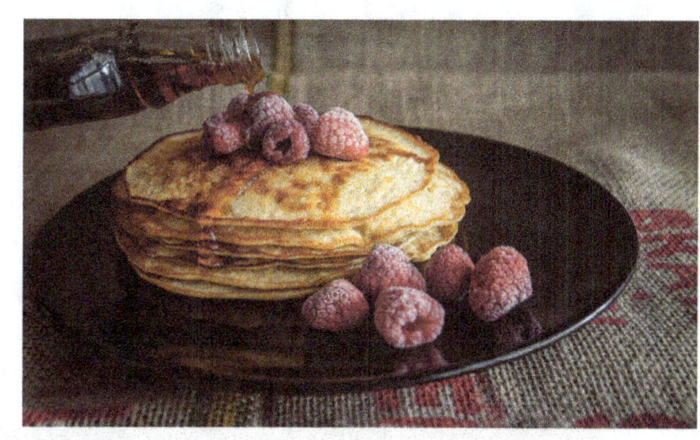

Ingredients

95g gluten free flour
1 tsp baking powder
3/4 tsp baking soda
Pinch of salt
1 large egg, lightly beaten
2 tsp butter, melted and cooled
230ml lactose free milk
100g raspberries
1 tbs olive oil

To serve:
'Live' natural yoghurt
Maple syrup
Extra raspberries

Directions

1. Whisk together flour, baking powder and baking soda.
2. Add a pinch of salt and set aside.
3. In large bowl, whisk together egg, butter and milk.
4. Add to flour mixture; stir just until combined. Fold in raspberries.
5. Heat a pan with 1 tbs of oil over moderately high heat.
6. Drop tablespoons of the batter onto the pan and cook for 2-3 minutes or until bubbles form on top.
7. Turn and cook for 1 minute on the other side.
8. Serve with a sprinkle of icing sugar, up to 2 tbs 'live' natural yoghurt and maple syrup

Fibre Power Oatmeal

Serves 1

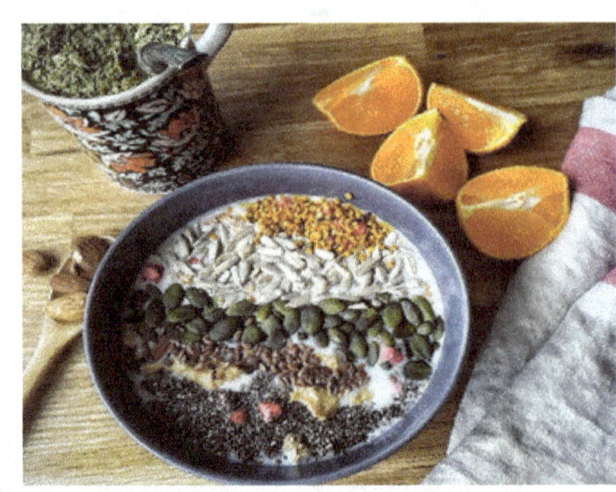

Ingredients

40g oats
200ml almond milk
1 tbs peanut butter
½ tbs chia seeds
½ tbs sunflower seeds
½ tbs pumpkin seeds
3 Brazil nuts

Pinch ground cinnamon, if desired
1 tbs low FODMAP granola (see recipe above)
1 tbs maple syrup
1 tsp dried cranberries

Directions

1. Place oats, milk and cinnamon in a small pot and place over medium heat and stir occasionally
2. Once thickened, put into a bowl and top with peanut butter, nuts, seeds, fruit and granola (in rows to make it look pretty!)

Low FODMAP Avo-Egg on Toast

Serves 1

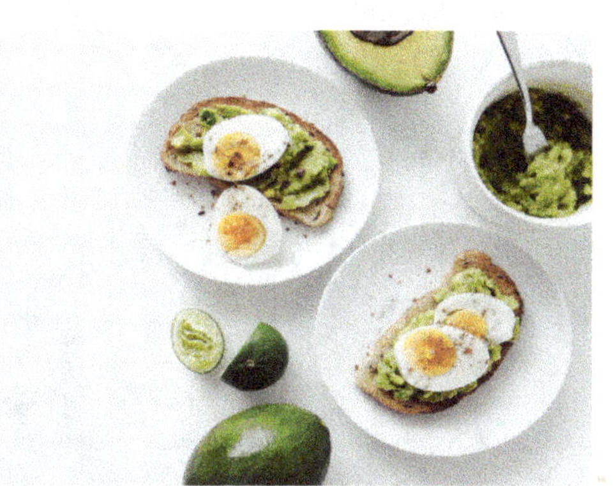

Ingredients

1/8 or 30g avocado
40g feta cheese
1 tsp lime juice
2 slices low FODMAP bread
Small pinch chili flakes
3 small baby vine tomatoes sliced

2 eggs
1tbs vinegar
20g pine nuts, toasted
Salt and pepper to taste

Directions

1.Place your avocado, feta, and lime juice in a small bowl and mash together with a fork until smooth.

2.Toast your bread and spread the avo mix onto toast and sprinkle with salt and chili flakes.

3. Top with tomatoes.

4. To begin poaching the eggs, break the two eggs into a ramekin or similar sized dish. Bring a small saucepan half filled with water and the vinegar to the boil, then lower the heat to a simmer. Stir the water in the pot to creates a funnel in the centre of the pot. Drop your eggs into the centre of the funnel and let it cook for 3-4 minutes, then remove it with the slotted spoon. Pat the eggs dry, and pop it on your toast.

5.Season with extra black pepper and sprinkle with toasted pine nuts, if desired, before serving straight away

Buckwheat Pancakes

Serves 2

Ingredients

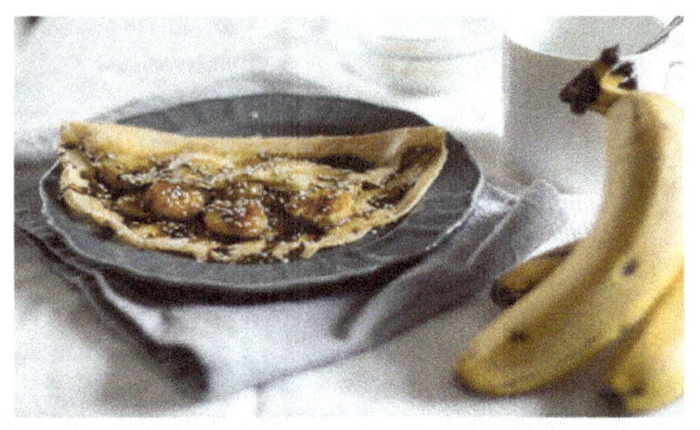

250ml lactose free milk
1 egg
Pinch salt
1 tsp olive oil
100g buckwheat flour
Butter for frying pancakes

Topping suggestions:
Banana
Toasted sesame seeds
1 tbs maple syrup
20g hazelnut spread

Directions

1. Place the milk, egg, salt and oil into a large bowl and mix well.
2. Sift the buckwheat flour into a separate bowl.
3. Gradually add the flour to the milk mixture, stirring constantly until a smooth batter is formed
4. Allow to rest for 30 minutes before cooking.
5. Add a small drop of oil to a hot pan, pour a large spoon of the mixture onto the pan and cook until air bubbles start to appear at the centre of the pancake.
6. Turn and cook for another 3-4 minutes, until nicely browned. Continue cooking the rest of the pancakes as above
7. Serve with favourite toppings

Cheesy French Toast

Serves 2

Ingredients

10 cherry tomatoes
1 tsp olive oil
1 tsp fresh or dried oregano
2 eggs
120ml lactose free milk
40g grated cheese

1 tsp ground cinnamon
Salt and black pepper to season
2 tsp olive oil
4 slices wholegrain gluten free bread

Directions

1. Heat oven to 220C. Mix tomatoes with oil and oregano and roast on a tray for approx. 15 minutes until skins pop.
2. Whilst tomatoes are cooking, break 2 eggs into a bowl and beat lightly with a fork. Stir in milk, cheese, cinnamon and season to taste.
3. Over medium-low heat, heat pan coated with the rest of the oil
4. Place a slice of bread, one at a time, into the egg mixture, letting the bread soak for a few seconds. Then carefully turn to coat the other side.
5. Transfer bread slices to pan, heating slowly until bottom of the bread slice is golden brown. Turn and brown the other side.
6. Serve the French toast with some roasted tomatoes on top.

Flourless Banana Pancakes

Serves 1

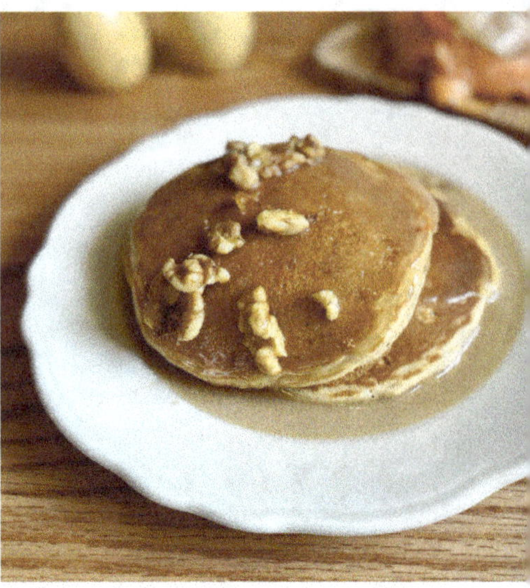

Ingredients

1 banana
1 tbs milled flaxseed
2 eggs
1 tsp vanilla essence
Pinch ground cinnamon
1 tbs butter
Toppings
Chopped pecans
Maple syrup

Directions

1. Beat the eggs, flaxseed, bananas, cinnamon and vanilla essence together until smooth
2. Melt a little butter in a frying pan.
3. Once it is bubbling, pour ½ the egg mixture into the pan.
4. Once it is set on one side, flip it over and cook on the other side.
5. Repeat with rest of mixture.
6. Serve with chopped pecans and a little drizzle of maple syrup, if desired

ALive & Kicking Strawberry Smoothie

Serves 2

Ingredients

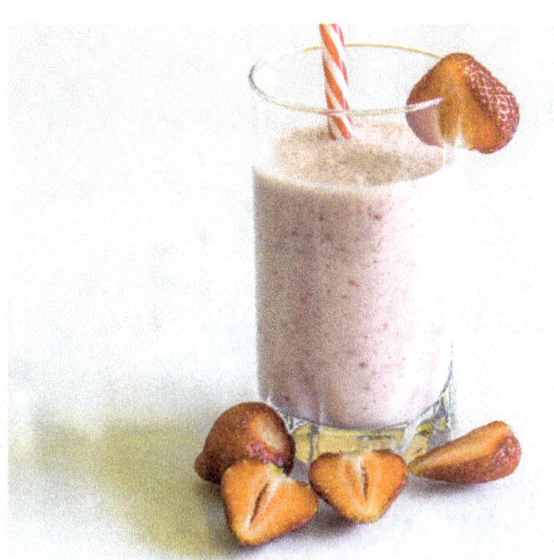

40g frozen strawberries
40g fresh or frozen pineapple
3 tbs hemp seeds
1 tsp ground psyllium husks
100g 'live' natural yoghurt
100ml water

Directions

1. Blend all ingredients until smooth and creamy
2. Serve in tall glass

Nutty Brekkie Bars

Serves ~12

Ingredients

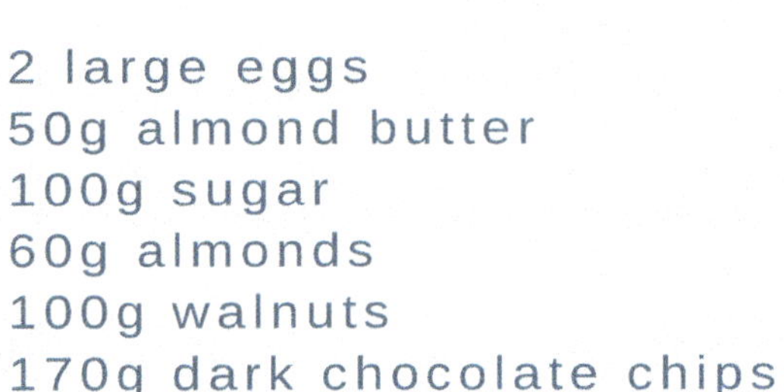

2 tbs olive oil
135g rolled oats
55g butter
70g gluten free flour
1 tsp cinnamon
½ tsp baking powder
½ tsp salt
1 tsp vanilla extract

2 large eggs
50g almond butter
100g sugar
60g almonds
100g walnuts
170g dark chocolate chips

Directions

1. Preheat oven to 180 degrees
2. Lightly grease a baking dish
3. Toast oats by placing olive oil in pan heat, then adding oats and stirring frequently. Place in a large bowl and let cool down.
4. Melt butter in separate pan and set aside
5. Add flour, cinnamon, baking powder, baking soda and salt to the cooled oats.
6. In a separate bowl add butter, eggs, almond butter, eggs and vanilla extract and mix together until smooth
7. Mix the dry oat mix into the wet ingredients
8. Then fold in the peanuts, walnuts and chocolate chips and mix
9. Pour the mixture into the lined backing tray and spread out evenly with spatula.
10. Bake for 18-20 minutes
11. Let bars cool down fully before slicing
12. Keep in an airtight container.

Egg Shakshuka

Serves 2

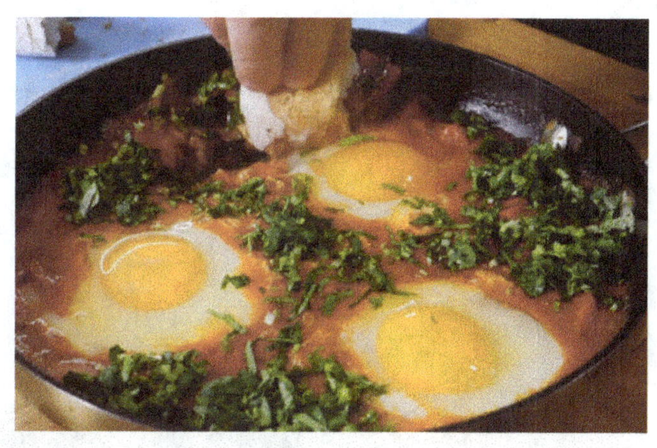

Ingredients

1 green pepper, deseeded & diced
2 large handfuls baby spinach
4 scallions, green tips only
1 tbs garlic infused oil
400g canned tomatoes
250ml low FODMAP vegetable stock
(see Miscellaneous recipe below)
1 tbs cornstarch
1 tsp paprika

1 tsp turmeric
1 tsp sugar or maple syrup
4 eggs
Salt and black pepper
2 tbs fresh coriander, chopped

Directions

1. Heat a large pan over medium-high heat. Add the garlic infused oil
2. Add the green pepper, tinned tomatoes and low FODMAP stock. Mix and allow the sauce to simmer for two minutes.
3. Dissolve the cornstarch in a small amount of warm water and stir through the sauce.
4. Add chopped spinach and green part of the spring onion. Allow the sauce to cook for another two minutes until it starts to thicken.
5. Add the spices and sugar. Stir and season with salt and pepper.
6. Turn the heat down to medium-low.
7. Crack the eggs into the tomato mixture, spacing them evenly around the pan. Cover and allow to simmer for 10 to 15 minutes until the eggs are cooked to your liking.
8. Sprinkle with coriander.
9. Serve with toasted low FODMAP bread

LUNCH

Making your FODMAP Life easy!

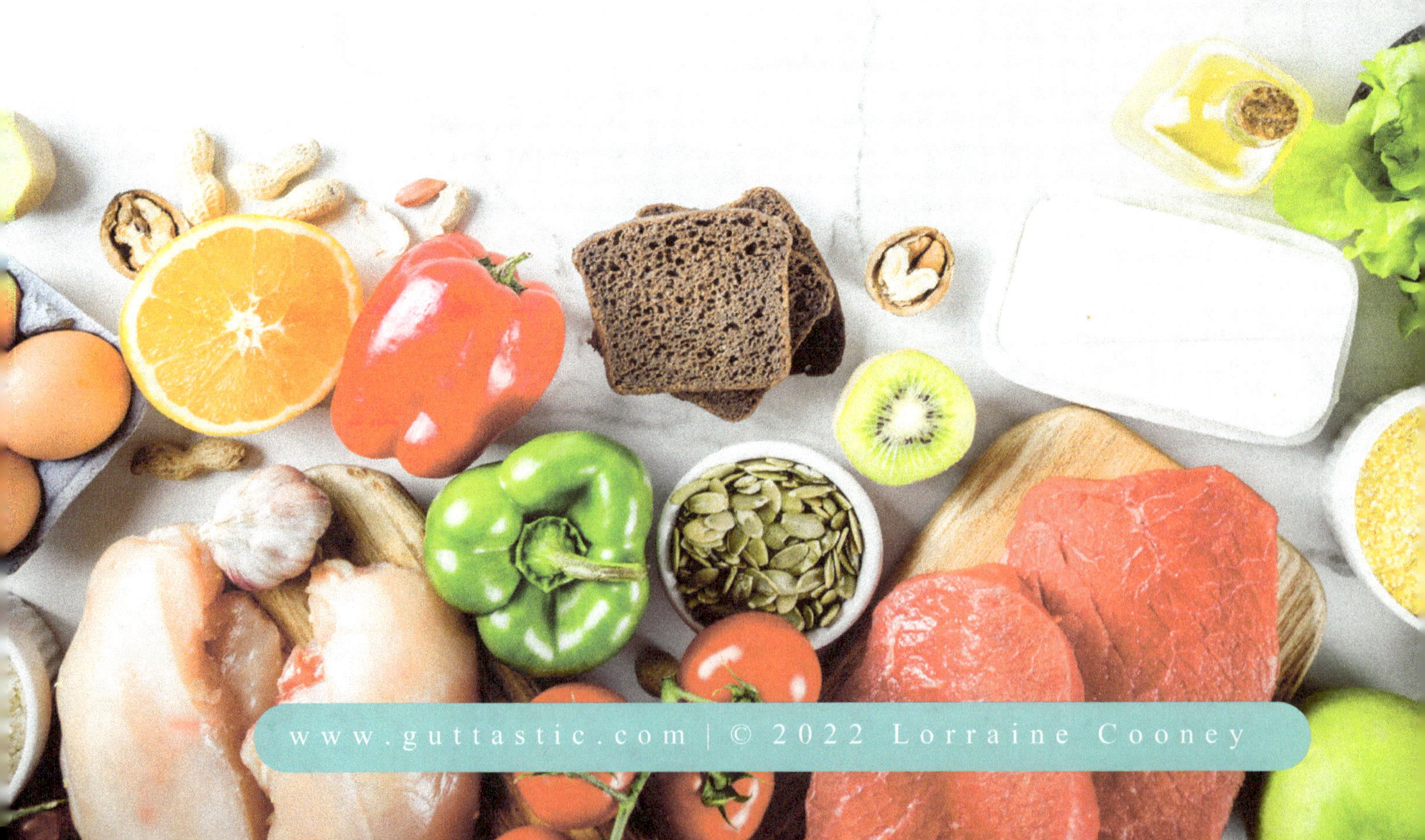

Minestrone Soup

Serves 3-4

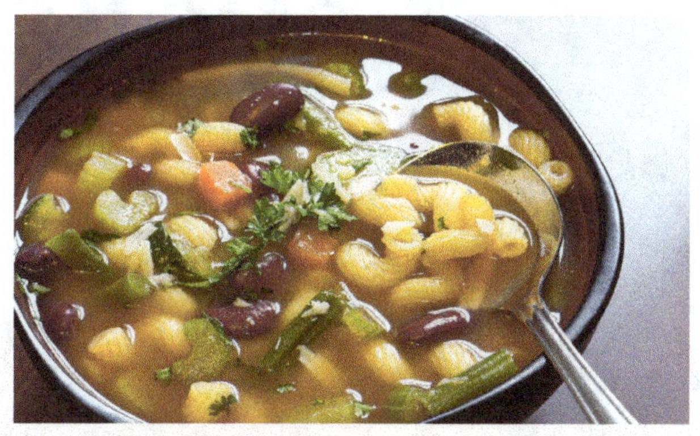

Ingredients

1 tbs garlic infused oil
2 medium carrots
8 tbs tomato puree
½ courgette
½ tsp dried oregano
½ tsp dried thyme
Salt and pepper to taste
1 can diced tomatoes
1L Low FODMAP stock (see recipe in Miscellaneous section)

200g gluten-free pasta
2 tsp freshly squeezed lemon juice
120g canned kidney beans, drained and rinsed (optional)
1 small bag kale
Serving suggestions:
Freshly grated Parmesan cheese
Freshly chopped parsley
Crusty Low FODMAP bread

Directions

1. Heat the oil in a large pan
2. Chop the carrot and courgette into bite sized pieces.
3. Add to the pan and cook for 5 minutes on medium heat
4. Add the dried herbs and cook gently for 1 minute
5. Add pasta, tomato puree, canned tomatoes, stock and lemon juice and bring to the boil
6. Lower to simmer and cook for 20 minutes.
7. Then add kidney beans, if using, and kale and cook for a further 5 minutes. Add more water if needed.
8. Remove from the heat
9. Serve with parmesan shavings, parsley and bread, as desired

Tuna & Artichoke Salad

Serves 1

Ingredients

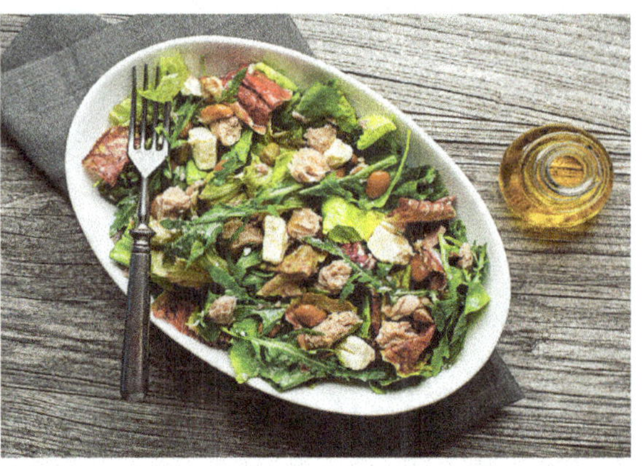

1 can tuna steak, drained
50g artichoke hearts quartered
30g feta
¼ cucumber, cut into chunks
2 handfuls mixed green
1 tbsp extra virgin olive oil
1 tbsp white wine vinegar
1/2 tbs maple syrup
Freshly ground black pepper

Directions

1. Mix the tuna, artichoke hearts, cucumber and feta and place on mixed greens in large bowl.
2. Whisk the oil, vinegar and maple syrup together then toss into the tuna mixture.
3. Season with black pepper before serving

Quinoa Tabbouleh

Serves 4

Ingredients

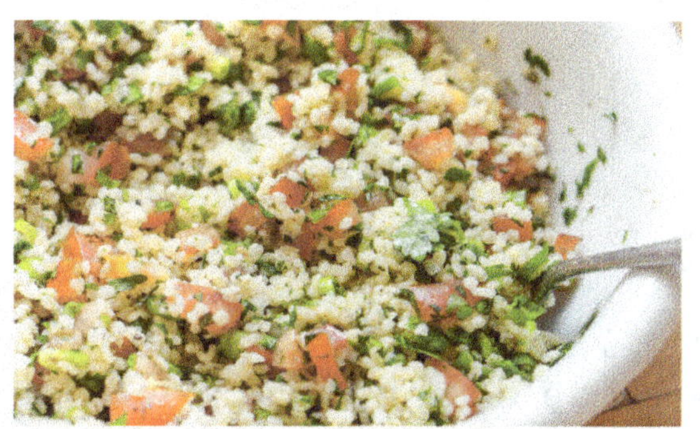

500ml vegetable stock
200g quinoa, rinsed well
4 eggs
2 tbsp garlic infused olive oil
10 small vine tomatoes, quartered
3 handfuls of spinach, thinly chopped
2 tbs lemon juice
Handful of fresh parsley
2 tbs sesame seeds
1 handful mint, chopped
Salt and pepper to taste

Directions

1. Place stock and quinoa in a large saucepan; bring to the boil. Reduce heat to low-medium; simmer for 15 minutes or until most of the stock is absorbed. Remove pan from heat and let cool.
2. Meanwhile, cook eggs in a small saucepan of boiling water for 7 minutes (can boil for 6 minutes if prefer softer yolk). Remove eggs immediately and cool under cold running water for 30 seconds.
3. Heat half the garlic infused oil in a pan over medium heat. Add spinach and stir until wilted. Add cooked quinoa, tomatoes, mint and lemon juice; season to taste.
4. Combine parsley, seeds and salt in a small bowl. Peel eggs; roll in parsley mixture.
5. Top quinoa tabbouleh with halved eggs.

Veg-tastic Omelette

Serves 2

Ingredients

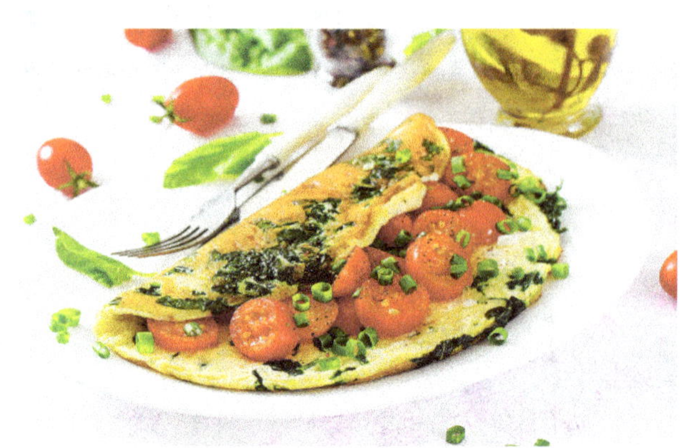

2 tbs olive oil
A pinch of asafoetida powder
1 tbs mixed dried herbs
1 red pepper, chopped into small pieces
6 cherry vine tomatoes, halved
4 eggs
Salt and black pepper to season
3 spring onions, green part only, thinly sliced
40g pitted black olives, sliced
Handful of spinach
Hanful of basil, chopped
60g feta cheese

Directions

1. Use a non-stick frying pan with lid
2. Heat 1 tbs olive oil in a frying pan and when getting hot add the asafoetida powder
3. Then add chopped peppers and tomatoes
4. Turn the heat right down & let it cook gently for approx. 10 minutes or until vegetables are tender. Mix halfway so they don't brown too much. Two minutes to the end add the spinach, green part of the spring onion and the olives. When cooked remove veg mix from the pan and set aside
5. Then break the eggs into a large bowl and whisk them lightly. Season well.
6. Put the frying pan back on the heat & pour the omelette mix into the frying pan and turning the heat down to its lowest setting immediately.
7. Intermittently draw the edge in gently with a palette knife. Cook the omelette for approx. 10-15 minutes uncovered.
8. Once it looks nearly set, add the veg mix into the middle and sprinkle the cheese on top. Flip over and serve straight away.

Kimchi Fried Rice

Serves 3

Ingredients

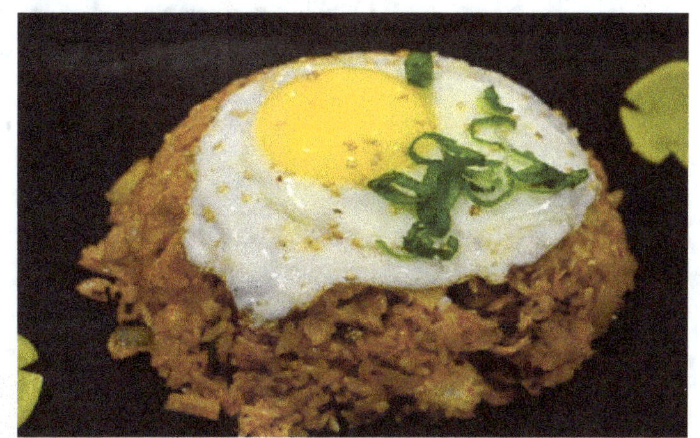

90g Kimchi
375g cooled boiled brown rice
200g oyster mushrooms
2 carrots, grated
2 large eggs
½ tbs sesame oil
1 tbs garlic infused oil
3 spring onions, green part only
1 tbs sesame seeds, toasted
1 tsp grated ginger
Nori strips, optional

Directions

1. Preheat a pan/wok and add garlic infused olive oil
2. Add kimchi & stir on low-medium heat until hot, about 2 minutes
3. Add carrots & mushrooms and cook for 3-4 mins
4. Reduce heat
5. Add rice and mix all ingredients
6. Add sesame oil & remove from pan/wok
7. Garnish with toasted sesame seeds, green part spring onion and strips of nori if desired
8. Lightly fry eggs and place on top

Peanut-Tofu Buddha Bowl

Serves 2

Ingredients

120g brown rice
1 cup water
Pinch of salt
75g spinach chopped
1 medium carrot, peeled and julienned
60g shredded red cabbage
90g edamame beans
3 tbsp olive oil
170g plain firm tofu

Peanut sauce
1 tbs sesame oil
2 tbs soya sauce
2 tbs maple syrup
2 tbs peanut butter
1 tbs water
To serve:
4 scallions, green part only
1 tbs sesame seeds

Directions

1. Place the rice in a sauce pan with boiling water and a pinch of salt. Reduce to a low heat and cook until all the water has been absorbed and the rice is cooked (about 8 minutes).
2. Drain and wrap the tofu with paper towel. Place a plate and a heavy object on top of the tofu and set aside for at least 15 minutes to drain faster
3. After pressing the tofu, cut into medium rectangular strips and season both sides with salt and pepper. In a hot grill pan, stir fry in olive oil for ~5 minutes until crispy and golden brown.
4. Whisk or blend together the ingredients for the sauce (sesame oil, soya sauce, maple syrup, peanut butter, water) until creamy and smooth.
5. Place the rice in two bowls, add the veg, tofu and edamame beans
6. Top with green onions and sesame seeds
7. Drizzle over the sauce before serving

Miso Roasted Veg with Lentils

Serves 2

Ingredients

2 medium parsnips, thinly sliced
2 medium carrots, thinly sliced
1 tbs poppy seeds
80g canned lentils (rinsed & drained)
90g baby spinach
I orange cut into segments
60g goat's cheese
Salt & pepper for seasoning

Marinade
2 tbs miso paste
1 tbs grated ginger
1 tbsp maple syrup
2 tsp orange zest
2 tbs olive oil

Directions

1. Preheat the oven to 180ºC.
2. Whisk or blend the miso paste, grated ginger, maple syrup, orange zest and olive oil. together.
3. Prep the carrots and parsnips and transfer into a single layer on a non-stick roasting tin.
4. Coat with half of the miso marinade and sprinkle with poppy seeds.
5. Roast in the oven for 20-25 minutes until the vegetables are tender and golden
6. Drain and rinse the lentils, then weigh the recommended single serving: 40g
7. Arrange the spinach onto the plates and top with the roast veggies, lentils, goats' cheese, and orange segments.
8. Then drizzle with remaining miso dressing.
9. Can be served both warm and cold

Kimchi Pancakes

Serves 2

Ingredients

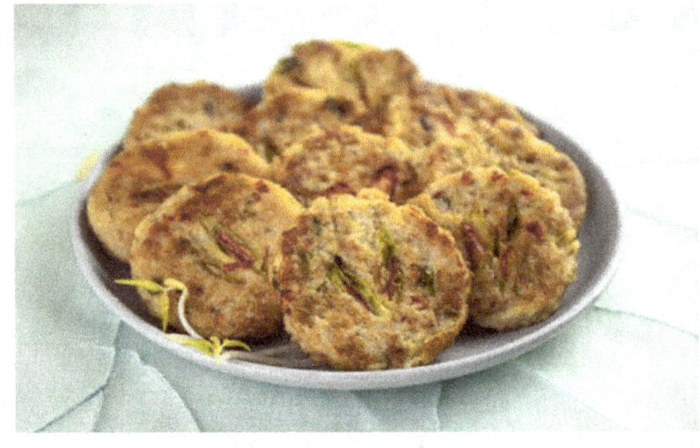

90g kimchi
100g rice flour
1 tsp turmeric
75ml lactose free milk
1 egg
1 tbs garlic infused oil
2 spring onion, green part only, chopped
1/2 red pepper, cut into thin strips
1 tbs toasted sesame seeds
50g coriander, chopped

Dipping Sauce
1 tbs soy sauce
1 tsp rice vinegar
1/2 tsp caster sugar
1 tsp fresh chives, optional

Directions

1. Mix together flour, turmeric, egg, milk, chopped scallions, red pepper and chopped kimchi until thoroughly combined. Season with salt and pepper
2. In a non-stick frying pan, add a spoonful of the pancake mix to create mini pancakes and cook on high heat for 1-2 minutes.
3. Turn heat to low/medium-low, cover and cook until crispy at the bottom and partially cooked on top (around 5-6 minutes).
4. Flip the pancakes over and continue cooking on the opposite side until crispy or place under the grill until pancake top is crispy and brown crispy.
5. While the pancake cooks, stir together the soy sauce, vinegar and caster sugar, and is using the fresh chives.
6. Serve the pancakes with the dipping sauce on the side. Garnish with sesame seends andfresh corander and serve straight away

Pasta Salad with Chickpeas and Feta

Serves 2

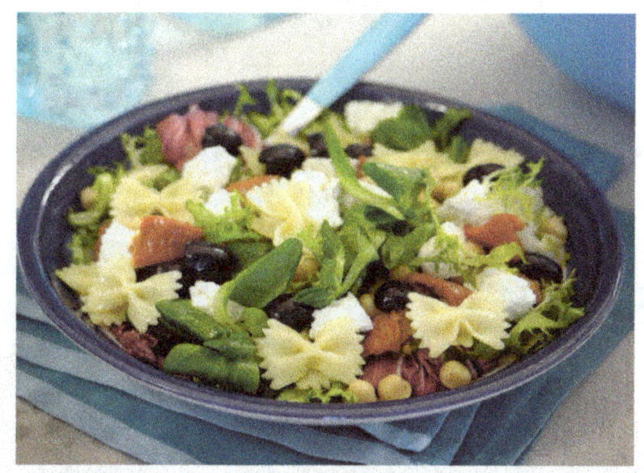

Ingredients

Pasta Salad
240g gluten free wholegrain pasta
160g tinned chickpeas, drained, rinsed thoroughly
150g feta cut into cubes
6 semi-sundried tomatoes
3 scallions, green parts only, chopped
250g cucumber, cut into quarter slices
2 handfuls mixed leaves
1 handful black olives

2 tbs fresh basil, finely chopped
2 tbs finely chopped fresh mint
2 tbs pine nuts
Salt and black pepper
Salad Dressing
60ml/ 4 tbs extra-virgin olive oil
15ml/1tbs apple cider vinegar
1 tsp Dijon mustard
Salt and black pepper

Directions

1. *Pasta Salad:* Bring a large pot of salt water to a boil and cook pasta until just al dente, about 10 minutes, until al dente. Drain and rinse with cool water to stop the cooking immediately.
2. *Dressing:* Shake the oil, vinegar and mustard together in a covered jar. Season to taste with salt and pepper
3. While pasta still a bit warm, add a few tablespoons of the dressing and toss to coat. Then allow pasta to cool to room temperature.
4. When cool, add the drained chickpeas, feta, tomatoes, cucumbers, black olives, scallions, mixed leaves and herbs
5. Dress with more salad dressing to your liking (may have leftovers!).
6. Season to taste. Can be served immediately or stored in airtight container

Thai Inspired Prawn & Rice Noodle Soup

Serves 4

Ingredients

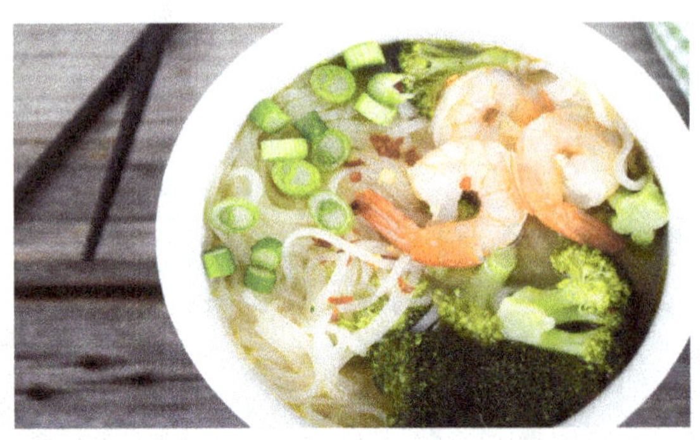

1 tbs garlic infused olive oil
1 tbs fresh ginger, grated
1L low FODAMP stock (see recipe in miscellaneous section)
1 can coconut milk
2 tbs fish sauce
4 heaped tsp dark brown sugar
2 tbs fresh lime juice

1 tsp turmeric
1 head broccoli, cut into single florets
300g thin rice noodles
300g king prawns, fresh or defrosted
To serve
Handful chopped fresh coriander
3 scallions, green parts, thinly sliced
Lime wedges

Directions

1. Cook the rice noodles according to the package instructions.
2. Heat the oil in a medium soup pot over medium-low heat.
3. Add the ginger and cook, stirring frequently, until softened, 3 to 5 minutes.
4. Add the broccoli, stock, coconut milk, fish sauce, brown sugar, lime juice, and turmeric; bring to a gentle simmer. Continue simmering, uncovered, for 5 minutes.
5. Add the prawns and cook for a few minutes (until prawns pink)
6. When ready to serve, taste the soup and adjust the seasoning to your liking.
7. Gently reheat the noodles in the microwave, if necessary.
8. Divide the noodles into serving bowls.
9. Ladle the prawn broth over top and sprinkle with coriander and scallions and lime wedges

Low FODMAP Falafel

Serves 6

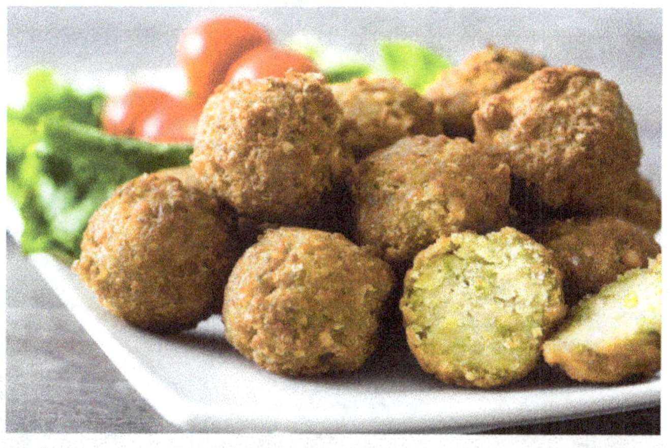

Ingredients

2 medium carrots, peeled & grated
240g chickpeas from can, drained & rinsed well
1 large lime, zest & juice
50g fresh parsley, stems removed
25g coriander leaves, stems removed
180g medium grain brown rice
1 tbs garlic infused oil
1 tsp paprika
1 tsp ground cumin

1 tsp ground coriander
4 tbs gluten free flour
Salt & pepper
1 tbsp olive oil
Sauce
2 tbs tahini
2 tbs lemon juice
1 tsp olive oil

Directions

1. Preheat the oven to 190ºC
2. *Prepare the falafel* Pre-cook the brown rice and cool. Place the rice, grated carrots, drained chickpeas, lime juice & zest, parsley, spices and garlic infused oil into a food processer. Blend until it forms a smooth paste - add 1-2 tbs water if too dry. Once it is well combined, stir through the gluten free flour. The texture should be mouldable
3. Line a baking tray and grease with olive oil.
4. Scoop out the falafel using a tablespoon and form into small patties. It helps to have wet hands as you form the patties.
5. Space the patties evenly on the tray. Brush with oil. Bake for about 12 minutes each side, until golden brown.
6. Alternatively, you can fry in a non-stick frying pan, cooking for 2-3 minutes on each side
7. Make the sauce by adding the tahini, lemon juice and olive oil together and mixing well
8. Serving tip: you can serve the falafels with the sauce with gluten free pita's, diced cucumber and tomatoes & rocket

Caprese Salad

Serves 2

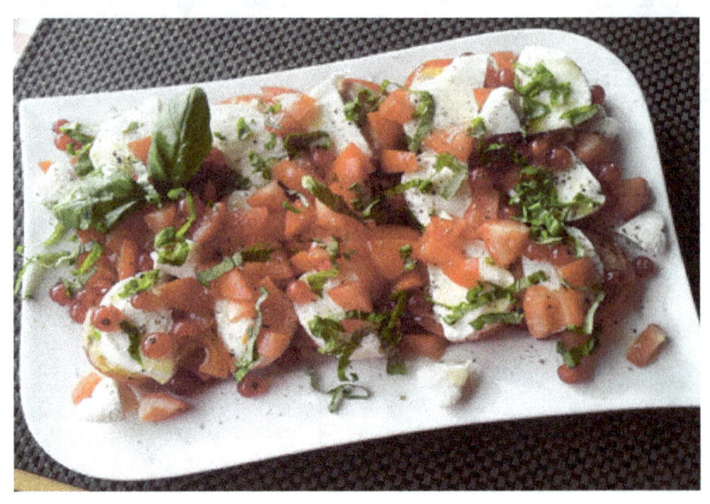

Ingredients

Salad
120g mozzarella ball
2 medium vine tomatoes
5 fresh basil leaves, finely chopped
2 tsp extra virgin olive oil
Salt and black pepper to season
Balsamic vinegar

Tomato salsa
2 medium vine tomatoes, finely diced
60 g pomegranate seeds
4 spring onion, green part only, finely chopped
5 fresh basil leaves, finely chopped

Directions

1. Cut the mozzarella and tomatoes into thin slices
2. Chop the basil leaves and mix with extra virgin olive oil in a small jug
3. To make the salsa, mix the tomatoes, pomegranate, spring onion and basil leaves together.
4. Layer alternating slices of mozzarella and tomatoes on the plate
5. Place a large spoonful of the salsa over the mozzarella
6. Pour extra some olive oil and drizzle with balsamic vinegar if desired

Rainbow Halloumi Wraps

Serves 2

Ingredients

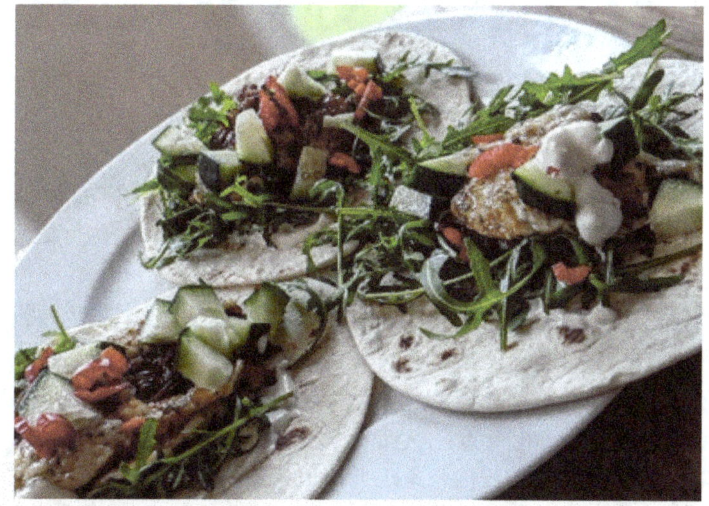

80g halloumi
60g baby pickled beetroot
¼ cucumber, sliced and quartered
1 tbs fresh mint
2 handfuls rocket
2 gluten free or corn tortilla wraps

Dressing
5 tbs natural yogurt
½ teaspoon Dijon mustard
3 tsp apple cider vinegar
2 tablespoons extra virgin olive oil

Directions

1. Slice the halloumi and grill on both sides for approx. 3-4 minutes until melting and browning
2. Slice the beetroot and cucumber
3. Discard the stalks from the mint and chop
5. Place all salad ingredients together into a bowel and mix.
6. Add all the dressing ingredients into a jar or jug and mix
7. Drizzle the dressing over the salad (may not need all of it)
8. Divide the salad between the tortilla wraps, then place the halloumi on top
9. Fold up the wraps and serve immediately

Gut Nourishing Diversity Bowls

Serves 2

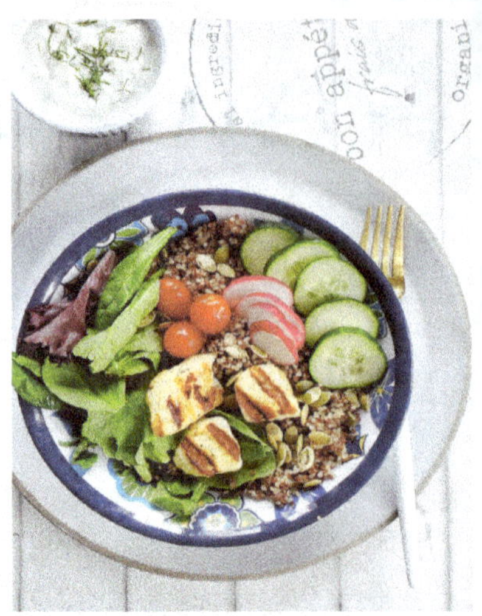

Ingredients

Customize!

Wholegrain: 120g brown rice OR quinoa OR millet

Protein: 120g chicken breast OR tofu OR 1 egg

2-3 Veg eg: cherry tomatoes, grated carrot, spinach, sliced red peppers, baby sweetcorn, rocket, cucumber

Pulses: 40g rinsed and drained canned chickpeas OR black beans or lentils

Seeds: 1 tbs sunflower seeds OR sesame seeds OR pumpkin seeds

Dressing:

3 tbsp olive oil extra virgin with

1 tbsp apple cider vinegar OR lemon juice OR balsamic vinegar

1 tsp mustard OR 1 tbs tahini or 1 tbs light soy sauce

Season to taste.

Directions

1. Choose your favourite grain and cook as per packet instruction

2. Choose favourite protein:

·Chicken: heat 2 tbs of olive oil in a pan over medium–high heat. Add the chicken, sprinkle some paprika and black pepper, cook each side for 5 minutes or until meat is cooked

·Egg: Cook the egg in a pan with boiling water for 10 minutes

·Tofu: drain and wrap with paper towel to dry out. Cut into squares and coat with salt and cumin. Wok fry until crispy and golden brown

3. Add 2-3 veg e.g. halved cherry tomatoes, grated carrots, shredded spinach, roasted peppers, rocket or baby sweetcorn

4. Drain and rinse one of the pulses and set aside 40g/2 tbs portion

5. Choose your favourite seed

6. Assemble bowls in a bowl or lunchbox. Cover the bottom with the grain. Add the protein, a vegetable and a pulse on top and sprinkle with the seeds.

7. For the dressing, in a small sealable jar or container, combine all the ingredients and shake until smooth.

8. Toss over the dressing before eating

9. You can enjoy the nourish bowl cold or slightly heated in the microwave

DINNER

Making your FODMAP Life easy!

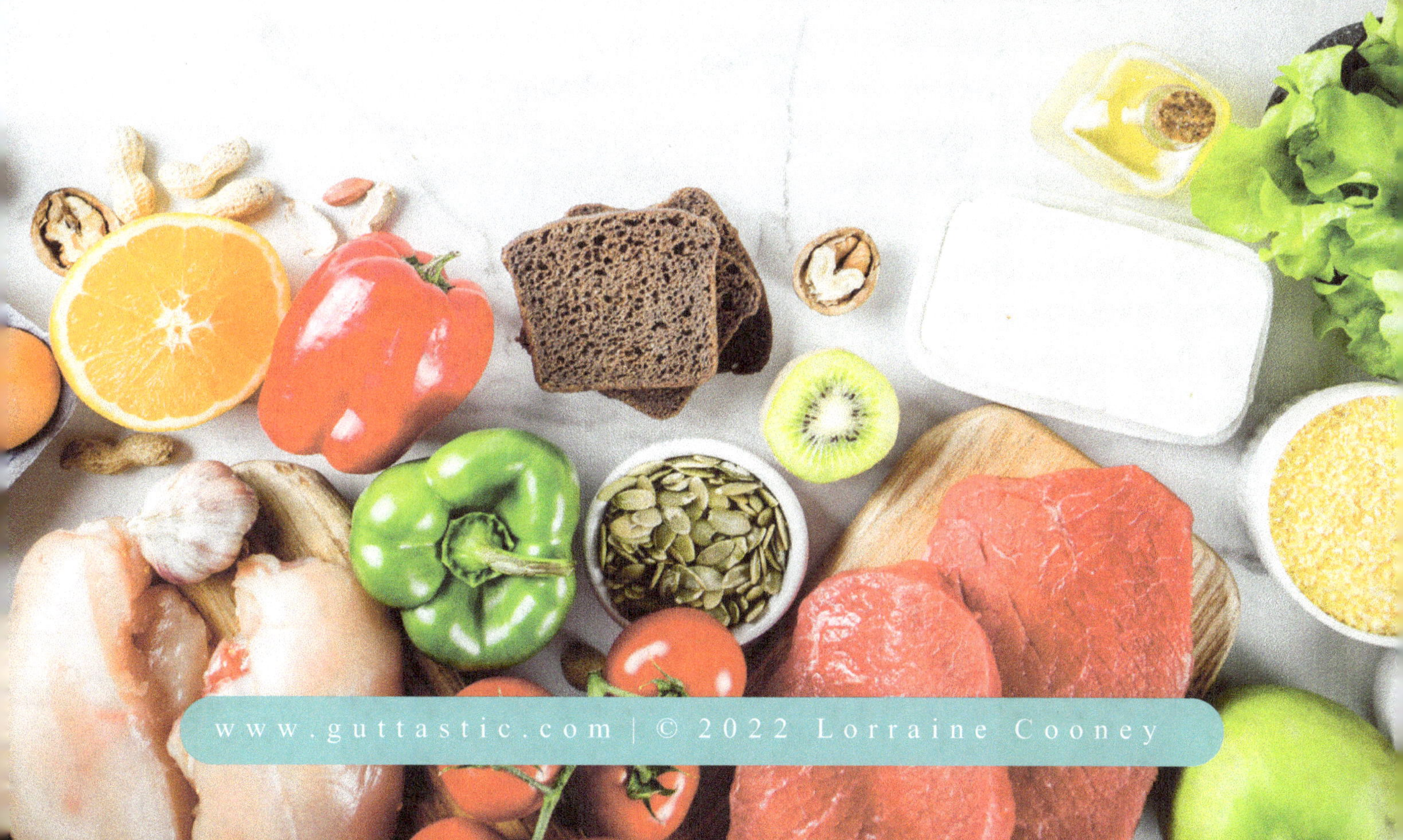

Chicken Fried Rice

Serves 4

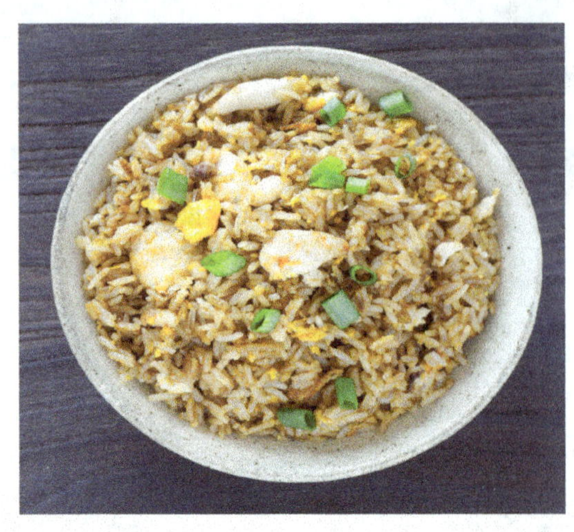

Ingredients

240g basmati rice
2 large eggs
Salt and freshly ground black pepper
1 tbs garlic infused olive oil
4 boneless, skinless chicken breast
fillets, cut into thin strips
2 tbs sesame oil

1 tbs curry powder
3 spring onion, the green
part only, thinly sliced, plus extra
for garnishing
200g courgette, sliced
200g green beans, sliced
2 tbs low sodium soy sauce

Directions

1 Cook the rice as per packet instruction

2 Beat eggs with a whisk in a bowl and season with salt and pepper.

3 Heat 1 tsp of the olive oil in a frying pan over medium heat and make a thin omelette
   using the beaten eggs.

4 Turn out onto a plate to cool and then coarsely chop into pieces. Set aside.

5 In a separate bowl, toss chicken strips with the sesame oil and season as desired.

6 Heat the remaining garlic infused olive oil and add the curry powder over high heat
   in a wok and stir-fry the prepared chicken strips until lightly golden, which will take
   about 2 to 3 minutes before removing from the wok.

7 Then add the green beans and courgette to the used wok and stir-fry for 3-4 minutes

8 Stir in the spring onion slices, cooked chicken & rice and sprinkle with soy sauce and
   mix all ingredients together.

9 Remove from heat and stir in chopped cooked egg.

10 Divide evenly among four bowls and, if desired, garnish with additional sliced green
   onions.

Sweet Potato & Feta Frittata

Serves 2

Ingredients

1 tbs garlic infused olive oil
4 eggs
150g of sweet potatoes, washed and peeled
3 handfuls baby spinach
70g of feta cheese
1 tsp thyme
1 tbs fresh chives (optional)
Salt & pepper for seasoning

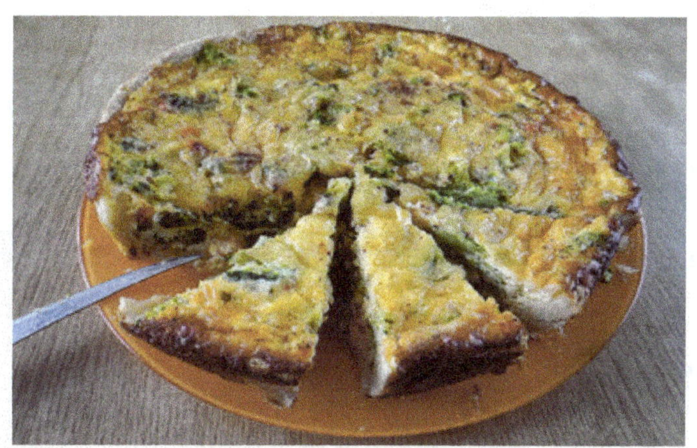

Directions

1. Preheat the oven to 200°C.

2. Cut the sweet potatoes into thin slices (not cubes) and steam until soft.

3. Meanwhile in a non-stick pan heat a teaspoon of oil and quickly sauté the spinach. Set them aside.

4. In a bowl, crumble the feta cheese and add the eggs and whisk everything together.

5. Add salt, pepper, thyme and finally the spinach.

6. Heat oil on the pan again, then add the chives and the sweet potatoes. Cook until golden brown and season with salt and pepper.

6. Pour the egg, feta and spinach mix over the potatoes.

8. Bake in a preheated oven for about 25 minutes or until the frittata is golden brown.

Pizza with 'Mix-Match' Toppings

Serves 4

Ingredients

Low FODMAP Pizza base
400g gluten-free flour
2 heaped tsp caster sugar
2 tsp baking powder
1 tsp salt
1 tsp xanthan gum
5 tbsp olive oil
Alternatively, you can buy a
pre-prepared base e.g. Dr. Schar
Low FODMAP Pizza sauce
2 tbsp olive oil
1 x 400g can chopped tomatoes
2 tbsp tomato purée
1 tsp sugar
2 handfuls fresh basil, chopped
Salt and pepper to taste

Mix and Match Toppings
Cheese e.g. mozzarella, feta, goats, cheddar
King prawns, pre-cooked
Sauteed oyster mushroom
Sliced tomato
Fresh or jarred roasted peppers
Black or green olives
Stir-fried aubergine cubes
Pineapple
Rocket
Red pepper flakes
Dried oregano
Fresh basil
Garlic infused oil

Directions

1 Heat the oven to 200 (with fan)

2 *To make the sauce* heat the oil in a small saucepan and add the chopped tomatoes, purée and sugar and bring to a gentle simmer. Cook, uncovered, for 25 - 30 mins or until reduced and thick, stirring regularly. Blend the sauce until smooth. Season to taste and stir through the basil. Allow to cool

3 *To make the pizza* mix the flour, sugar, baking powder, salt and xanthan gum in a large bowl. Make a well in the centre and pour in 250ml warm water and the olive oil. Combine quickly with your hands, to create a thick, wet, paste-like texture, adding an extra 20ml warm water if the dough feels a little dry. Store in an airtight container or covered bowl in the fridge for up to 24 hours before using.

4 When ready to use, lightly flour two baking trays. Split the dough into two and flatten with rolling pin on the sheets.

5 Finish the bases with a thin layer of the sauce and add your desired toppings

6 Place the baking sheets in the oven & cook for 8 -10 mins, until crisp around the edges.

Spaghetti Bolognese

Serves 4

Ingredients

500g lean beef mince
¼ tsp asafoetida powder
1 carrot, diced
½ red pepper, diced
2 tsp garlic infused olive oil
400g tin of tomatoes
2 tbs tomato puree
1 tbs balsamic vinegar
¼ tsp cinnamon
2 tsp dried Italian herbs
100g gluten-free spaghetti
60g Parmesan shavings
Salt and pepper, to taste

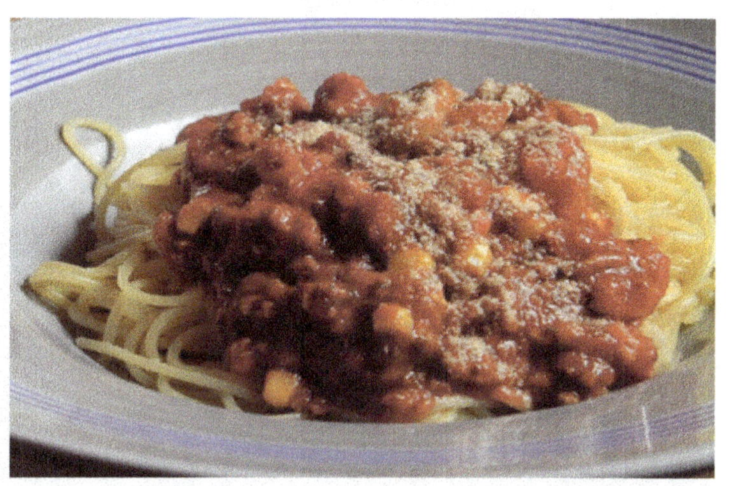

Directions

1. Heat garlic infused olive oil in a pan and add the asafoetida powder. Add carrot and pepper and cook until soft.
2. Add beef mince, and cook until browned, approx. 10 minutes
3. Add the tinned tomatoes, tomato puree, herbs, cinnamon, balsamic vinegar and season with salt and pepper.
4. Mix well and cook for 30min, or until sauce has reduced
5. Meanwhile, cook pasta according to direction.
6. Place the pasta in the bowls and top with Bolognese sauce
7. Sprinkle with parmesan and extra black pepper as desired

Ginger & Soy Salmon

Serves 2

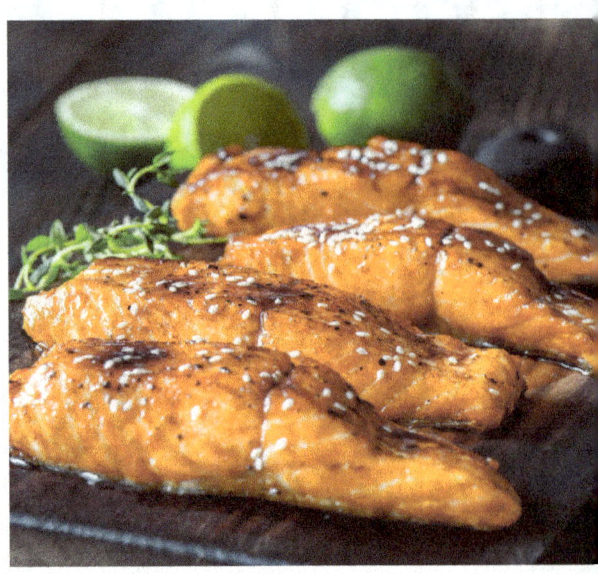

Ingredients

2 x 150g salmon fillet
2 tbs soya sauce
1/2 tbs oyster sauce
1 tsp grated ginger
1 tbs maple syrup
1 tbs garlic infused oil
1 head Bok choy, sliced in half lengthways
1 handful of green beans, topped and tailed
1 spring onion, sliced (green part only)
120g brown basmati rice

Directions

1. In a large Ziploc plastic bag, add the salmon, soya sauce, oyster sauce, ginger and maple syrup
2. Close the bag and shake contents to roughly coat the salmon. Marinate salmon in the fridge for as long as possible, ideally over 1 hour or overnight.
3. When ready to start, soak, rinse and cook rice as per packet instruction
4. Heat BBQ or grill to medium, and grease lightly with garlic oil. Place the salmon on the grill/pan (skin side down if using a fillet)
5. Cook for 5-6 minutes, or until skin becomes crisp. Flip and cook for another 3-4 minutes, or until the salmon is cooked to your liking
6. Meanwhile, heat the garlic infused olive oil in a wok and add the Bok choy, green beans, until soft, approx. 5-6 minutes, adding the spring onions near the end
7. Serve salmon with vegetables and basmati rice

Pasta with Prawns

Serves 4

Ingredients

240g gluten free pasta
2 tbs garlic infused olive oil
135g baby corn
1 red pepper, sliced
15 mange touts
450g pre-cooked king prawn
150ml white wine
2 heaped tbs tomato purée or paste
1 lemon. juice and zest
2 tbs fresh basil
2 tbs fresh parsley

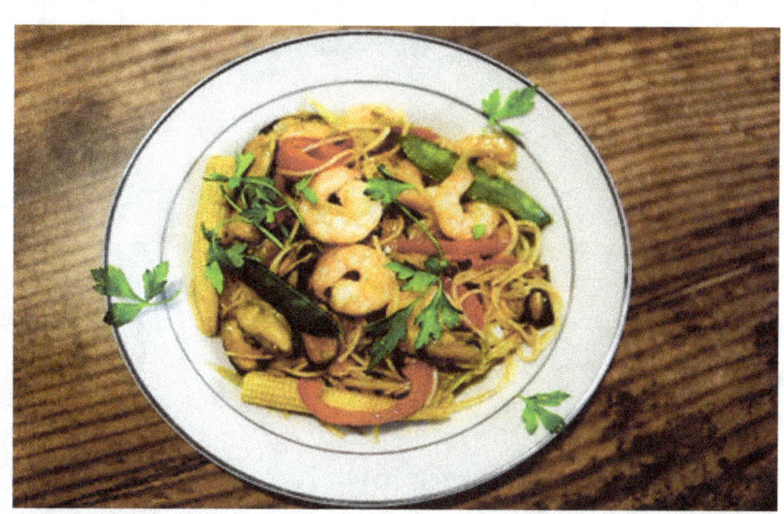

Directions

1. Cook pasta in a saucepan of salted boiling water until al dente. Drain.
2. While pasta is cooking, heat garlic infused olive oil in pan and add the baby corn, red pepper and mange tout and cook for about 5-8 minutes until veg are softening
3. Add the white wine and tomato purée, and simmer for a couple of minutes
4. Add prawns, basil and parsley and a squeeze of lemon juice to tomato sauce and cook for 1 minute. Remove from heat.
5. Grate the zest of the lemon.
6. Divide pasta among bowls. Top with prawn sauce and serve with lemon zest
7. Season to taste with sea salt and black pepper

Moroccan Chicken with Yoghurt Dip

Serves 4

Ingredients

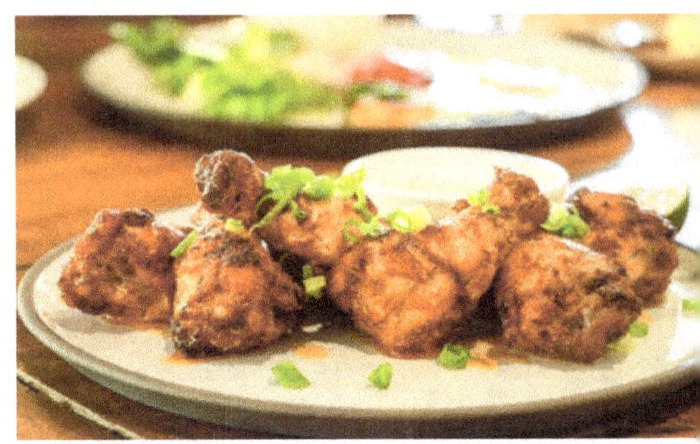

50g garlic infused oil
2 tsp ground paprika
1 tsp ground cumin
½ tsp salt
½ tsp ground coriander
½ tsp ground cinnamon
½ tsp ground turmeric
¼ tsp ground ginger
⅛ teaspoon cayenne pepper, optional
500g chicken thighs (or breasts)

Yoghurt Dip
200g Greek or plain lactosefree yoghurt
1 tbs fresh lemon juice
1 tbs chopped fresh mint
1 tbs chopped fresh coriander
1 tbs maple syrup
¼ tsp freshly ground black pepper

Directions

1. In a small bowl, whisk together all ingredients except chicken. Transfer mixture to a Ziploc bag or container with a lid. Add chicken and mix to coat. Seal and marinate the chicken in the refrigerator for at least an hour but ideally 8 hours.
2. When ready to eat, preheat grill on high. Remove chicken from marinade, discarding any leftover marinade.
3. Grill chicken thighs for 6-8 minutes per side or until cooked through
4. To make the dip, simply mix all the ingredients together and chill until ready to serve with chicken.

Halloumi Tray Bake

Serves 4

Ingredients

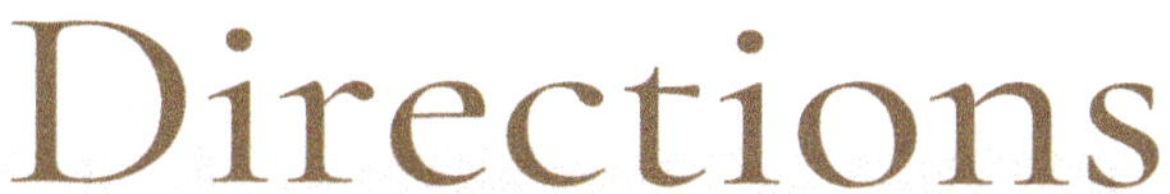

750g baby new potatoes, halved
4 tbsp garlic infused olive oil
1 large aubergine, chopped into cubes
1 large red pepper, deseeded and sliced into strips
200g broccoli florets
250g cherry tomatoes
160g halloumi, thinly sliced
4 scallions, green part only, chopped
Small bunch basil

Directions

1. Heat oven to 160C
2. Put the potatoes in a large roasting tin. Pour over 2 tbsp garlic infused olive oil and roast in the oven for about 10 mins.
3. Add the aubergine, red pepper and broccoli. Drizzle with another 2 tbsp oil, then roast for a further 15 mins until everything is softening
4. Then add the tomatoes and halloumi slices on top of the potatoes and veg and cook for another 10-15 minutes until the cheese is melting and browning (keep an eye on it).
5. Roughly tear the basil leaves and scatter over the halloumi bake just before serving.

Coconut Fish Curry

Serves 4

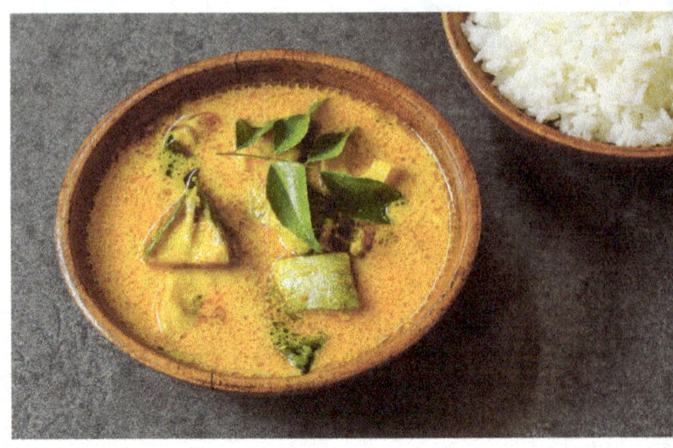

Ingredients

1 tbsp garlic infused olive oil
½ tsp asafoetida powder
Thumb-sized piece ginger, finely grated
1 tsp shrimp paste
1 small red chilli, shredded (optional)
2 lemongrass stalks, split, then hit with a rolling pin
1 tsp medium curry powder
1 tsp cumin
1 tsp garam masala
1 tbsp light muscovado sugar

3 medium tomatoes
1-2 heads baby Bok choy
Handful coriander, stems finely chopped
400g can coconut milk
450g skinless hake fillets, cut into rectangles
2 tbs fresh lime juice
Cooked basmati brown rice, to serve

Directions

1. Heat the oil in a frying pan
2. On low-medium hear, stir in the ginger, shrimp paste, chilli (if using) and lemongrass, and cook for 2 mins.
3. Add the curry powder, garam masala, cumin and sugar stirring.
4. When everything starts to clump together, add chopped tomatoes, and cook for 4-5 minutes
5. Then add the coriander stems, coconut milk and 2 tbsp water.
6. Bring to a boil, then lower the heat and cook for 15 minutes (low simmer).
7. Then add the fish and Bok choy. Cook for 5-6 minutes over low heat, until the hake is just cooked and flaking.
8. Then stir in the freshly squeezed lime juice and serve with cooked rice
9. Optional: sprinkle with chopped coriander and black cumin seeds

Chicken and Lentil Stew

Serves 4

Ingredients

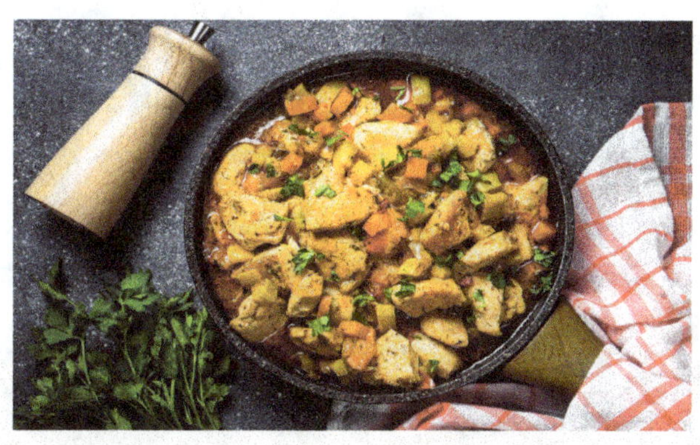

4 medium chicken breasts
2 tbs garlic infused oil
½ red pepper, cored and cut into thick strips
½ yellow pepper, cored, chopped
2 tsp ground coriander
1 tsp dried oregano
1 tsp smoked paprika

1 can chopped tomatoes
240ml low FODMAP stock (see recipe in Miscellaneous section)
100g tinned lentils, rinsed, and well drained
10 scallions, green parts only, chopped
1 tbs chopped flat-leaf parsley
Salt and pepper

Directions

1. Chop chicken into chunks and season the chicken on all sides with salt and pepper.
2. Add oil to large pan and cook chicken on both sides over low-medium heat and cook for about 10 minutes then remove from pan.
3. Add pepper strips to re-oiled pan and sauté over low-medium heat for a few minutes or until beginning to soften, then stir in the coriander, oregano and smoked paprika and about 1 minute, combining everything well.
4. Add the canned tomatoes and stock and put the chicken back into the pan, cover and bring to a boil
5. Simmer for about 25 minutes and then add the lentils and scallions and cook for a fruther few minutes..
6. Season and garnish with parsley before serving.

Beetroot & Goats Cheese Risotto

Serves 4

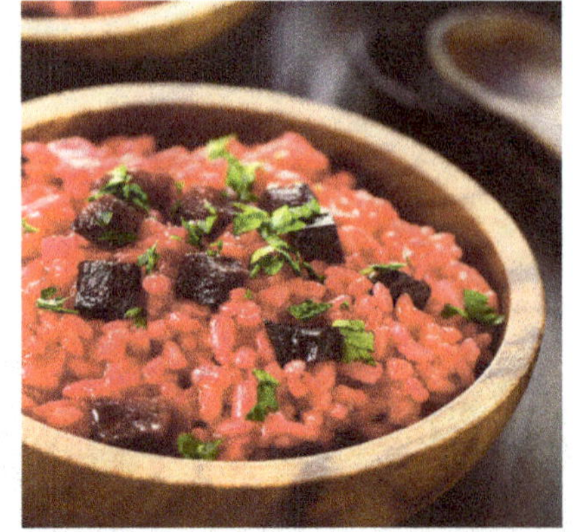

Ingredients

1L Low FODMAP friendly stock (see recipe in miscellaneous section)
300g pickled baby beetroot, chopped
2 tbs garlic infused oil
1 tbs butter
A pinch of asafoetida powder
40g celery, finely chopped
1 carrot, finely diced.
300g Arborio rice

250ml dry white wine
150g goat's cheese
50g freshly grated parmesan
Small bunch fresh parsley, finely chopped
Salt and pepper to season
Handful of kale leaves, trimmed, washed and dried

Directions

1. Heat the stock in a saucepan and keep on low heat whilst cooking the risotto
2. In a separate saucepan, heat the garlic infused oil and butter and add the asafoetida powder, followed by the diced celery and carrot and cook slowly for about 10-15 minutes until soft
3. Add the rice and stir for 1-2 minutes on medium heat.
4. Then add the wine and wait until it has been absorbed into the rice
5. Begin adding the stock one ladle at a time as it is absorbed into the rice and stir frequently. It takes 15-20 minutes to cook the rice.
6. The ideal risotto is soft but still has a bite! Use extra boiling water if you run out of stock.
7. Then 3/4 of the chopped beetroot and stir through the parsley
8. Remove from the heat and add the crumbled goats cheese, grated parmesan cheese and black pepper. Stir.
9. Garnish with remaining beetroot and kale

Tasty Tofu Stir Fry

Serves 4

Ingredients

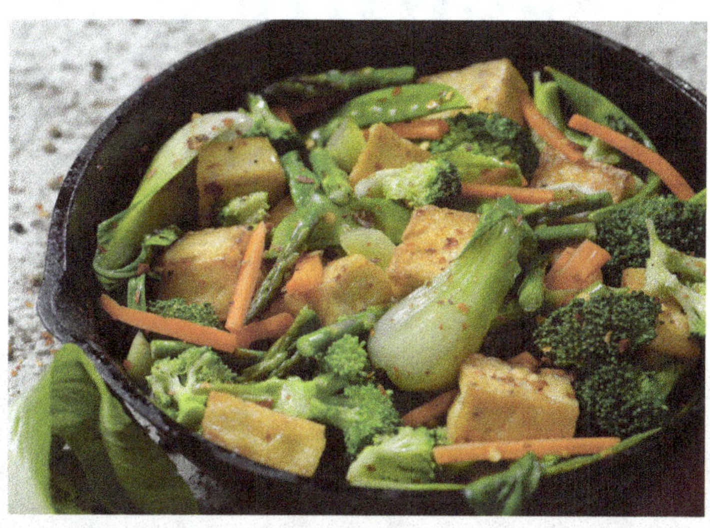

Stir-fry
2-3 tbs garlic infused oil
6 spring onion green part only, sliced
2-3 medium carrots, cut into thin slices
130g baby corn, cut in half lengthways
1 head of broccoli, cut into florets
1 head Bok choy, sliced
Thumb size ginger, thinly sliced
500g firm tofu
½ ime
Soba noodles
Black pepper

Sauce
2 tbs soya sauce
2 tsp sesame oil
2 tbs maple syrup

Garnish
Scallions, green part, chopped
Toasted sesame seeds

Directions

1. Stir together the soya sauce, sesame oil and maple syrup in a bowl, then set aside.
2. Place a wok over a high heat.
3. Pat the tofu dry and cut the tofu into cubes, then place in a bowl and dust with the cornflour and a pinch of sea salt and black pepper.
4. Place a wok over a medium- high heat. Add and heat the garlic infused oil.
5. Fry the tofu until golden and crisp, then scoop it out of the pan with a slotted spoon and set aside on a plate lined with kitchen paper.
6. Re-oil the wok and add the ginger, broccoli, courgette and carrot slices and stir-fry for a further 4 minutes.
7. Add the tofu back in and squeeze in the juice from half the lime and the green part of spring onion and add a splash of soy sauce
8. Prepare the noodles
9. Then serve the tofu-vegetables mix with soba noodles, and top with the extra scallions and toasted sesame seeds

Peanut Quinoa Stew

Serves 4

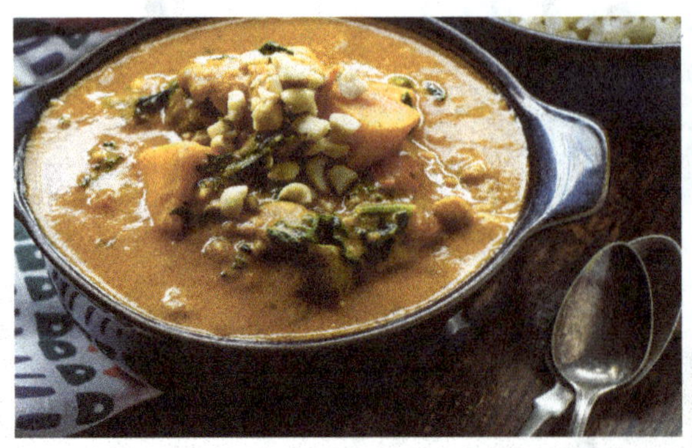

Ingredients

1 tbs garlic infused olive oil
Thumb size ginger, grated
1 tsp ground coriander
1 tsp ground cumin
1 tsp dried oregano
1 red pepper, diced
200g sweet potatoes, peeled, cut into cubes
1 tin chopped tomatoes
4 cups low-FODMAP vegetable stock
(or water)

150g quinoa, rinsed and drained
120g smooth peanut butter
150g fresh spinach, chopped
Juice of 2 small lemons
Salt & pepper, to taste
To serve:
Fresh coriander, chopped
Peanuts, crushed or whole

Directions

1. In a large pot, heat oil over medium heat, add the ginger, and cook for 3-5 minutes stirring frequently.
2. Add the quinoa, sweet potatoes, tinned tomatoes, dried spices, oregano and stock/liquid, and bring to a boil.
3. Reduce heat and simmer for 15 minutes, or until sweet potatoes are fork tender.
4. Turn off heat and stir in the peanut butter, and finish with the spinach and lemon juice.
5. Soup will thicken upon cooling. Season with salt & pepper to taste.
6. Serve in individual bowls with extra peanuts

Saag Paneer

Serves 4

Ingredients

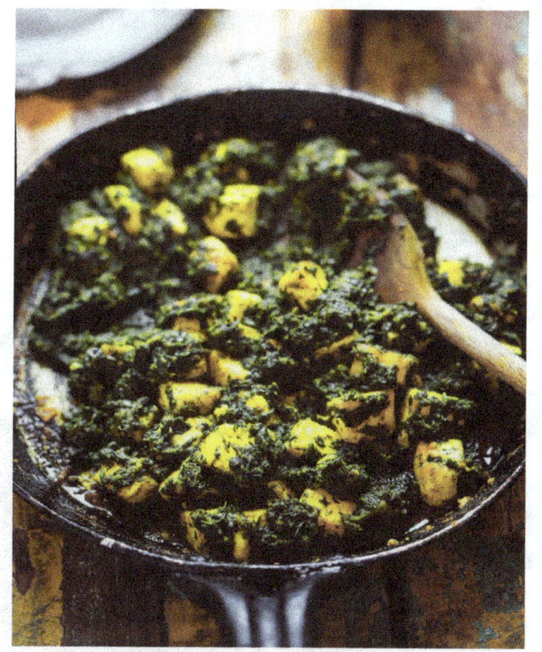

1 tbs garlic infused olive oil
½ teaspoon asafoetida
1 heaped tsp mustard seeds
1 tsp garam masala
1 tsp turmeric
1 small red chilli, de-seeded and finely chopped
A small thumb sized piece of ginger, peeled and grated
160g paneer cheese, cut into 3cm cubes
300g baby spinach
A handful of coriander leaves roughly chopped (optional)

Directions

1. Heat the oil in a medium pan and add the asafoetida followed by the mustard seeds
2. Once the mustard seeds start to pop, add the garam masala, turmeric, chilli and ginger and stir for a minute
3. Add the paneer cubes and cook over medium heat for around 8 minutes, tossing the pan so they become golden all over.
4. Then add the spinach to the pan and cook for a few minutes until it has wilted, sprinkle over the chopped coriander then serve

SNACKS

Making your *FODMAP* Life easy!

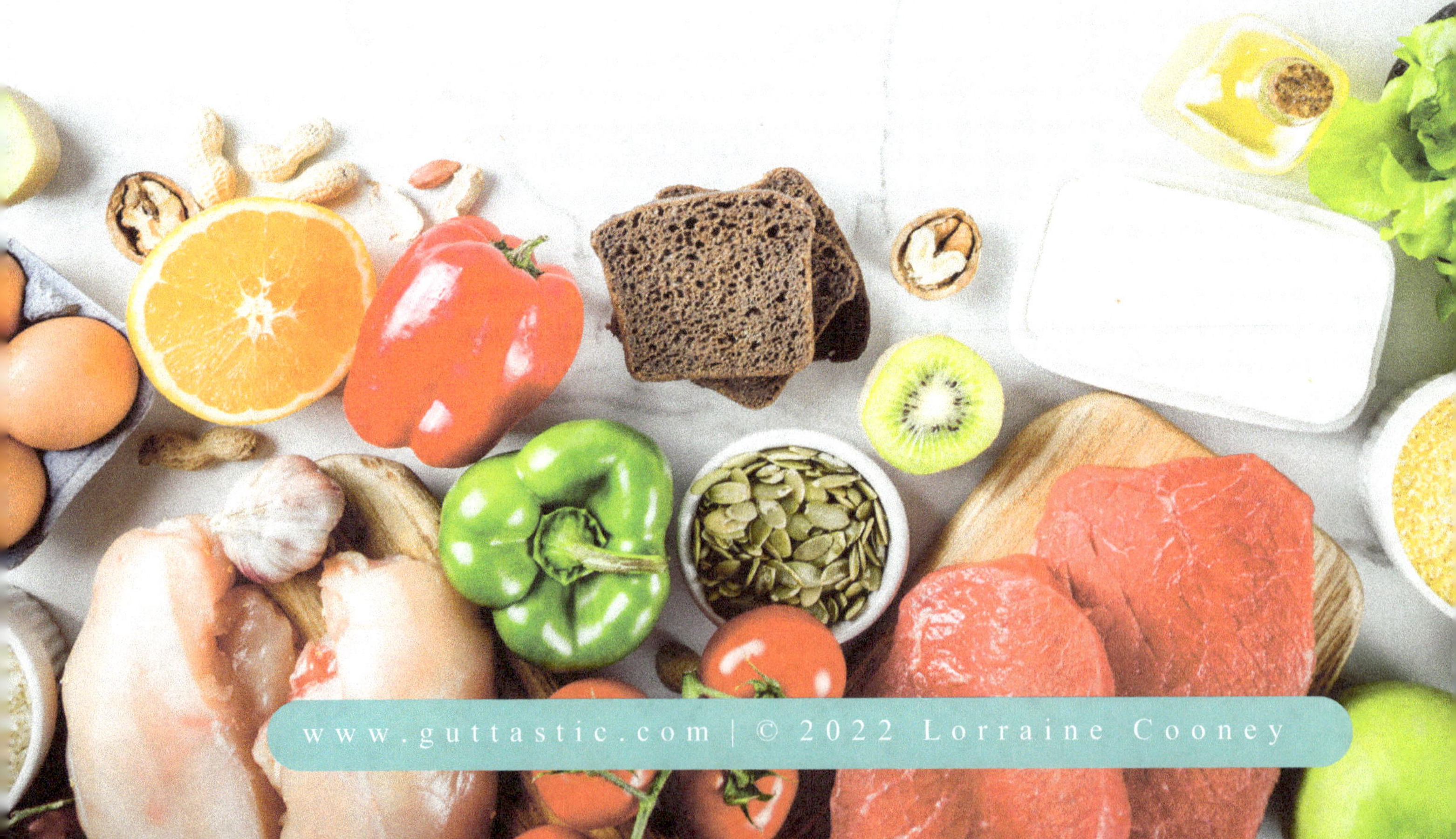

Frozen Banana Bites

Serves 4

Ingredients

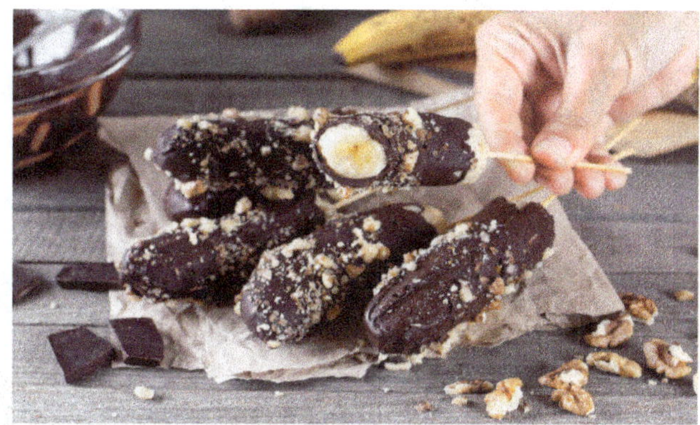

4 bananas
60g almond butter
100g dark chocolate
Crushed walnuts to roll

Directions

1. Peel and slice the banana in half

2. Place some almond butter on one inner side and place the another slice of banana on top - like a sandwich!

3. Place a small lolly pop stick or toothpick through the 'sandwich', squeeze together and place in the freezer for an hour

4. When the banana is frozen remove from the freezer.

5. Place the chocolate in a microwave safe bowl and melt

6. Swirl each banana lolly in the chocolate until it is coated then roll in crushed walnuts

7. Freeze again until the chocolate sets, about another hour

8. Keep in the freezer until required!

Energy Balls

Serves 12 balls

Ingredients

50g Low FODMAP mixed nuts* (e.g. walnuts, Brazil nuts, pecans, macadamias)
50g mixed seeds (e.g. sunflower, pumpkin, sesame)
40g oats
1 tsp ground cinnamon
4 tbs Greek yoghurt
60g natural peanut butter
2 tbs maple syrup
1 tsp vanilla extract

Directions

1.Put the nuts and seeds in the food processor and blend until coarse.
2.Add the oats and blend again
3.Then add the cinnamon, yoghurt, peanut butter, maple syrup and vanilla extract and blend thoroughly.
4.Mixture should combine to form balls easily.
5.Roll mixture into balls approximately the size of a walnut.
6.Place in the freezer for one hour before eating.
8.Can be eaten frozen or room temperature, and stored in the fridge for up to 4 days.

Kween Kiwi Smoothie

Serves 1

Ingredients

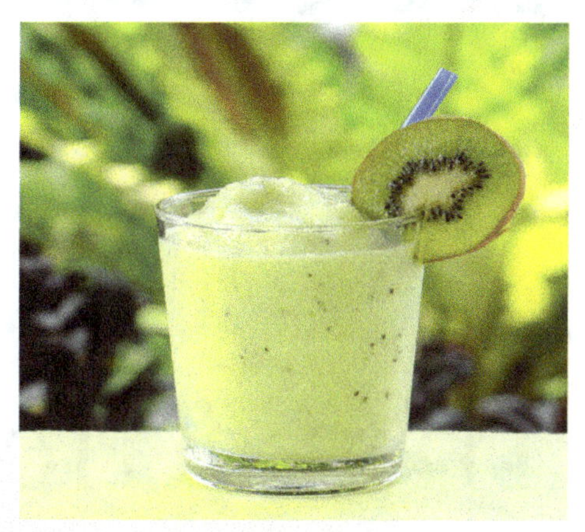

2 kiwis, with skin option (more fibre with skins on!)
200ml of lactose free milk
Handful of spinach
½ tsp fresh ginger, finely grated
1 tsp maple syrup, optional
Couple of ice cubes

Directions

1. Top and tail the kiwi fruit and cut into slices
2. Whiz the kiwi fruit with the remaining ingredients in a blender for 30 seconds and pour into a tall glass.
3. Sweeten with a little maple syrup if desired

Beet-ilicious Smoothie

Serves 1

Ingredients

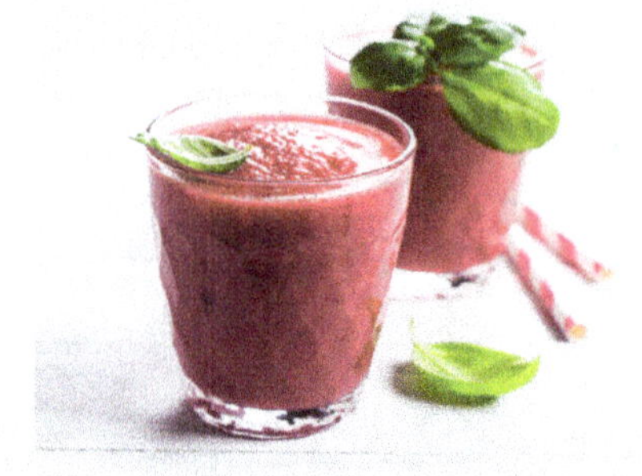

4-5 baby pickled beetroots
1/2 cup frozen raspberries
2 tsp chia seeds
Handful fresh spinach
150g non-dairy live coconut yoghurt
Ice cubes
A few basil leaves to serve

Directions

1. Blend all ingredients for 30 seconds and pour into a tall glass.
2. Use a splash of water if too thick
3. Decorate with some basil leaves

Trail Mix

Serves 6

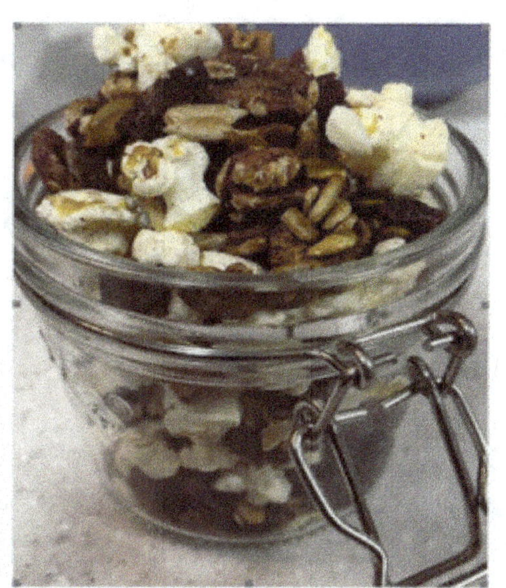

Ingredients

130g pecans
60g pumpkin seeds
60g sunflower seeds
30g salted popcorn
60g dried cranberries
45g dark chocolate, chopped
tsp cinnamon
2 tbs maple syrup

Directions

1. Combine pecans & seeds with maple syrup, mix well
2. Spread out evenly on baking tray and bake in oven for 10 mins at 170 degrees C
3. Let nuts and seeds cool completely, at least 10 minutes
4. When cool add popcorn, cranberries, and dark chocolate
5. Mix well
6. Sprinkle with cinnamon
7. Will last up to 4 weeks in airtight container or food bag

EspressoTahini Snack Balls

Serves 6

Ingredients

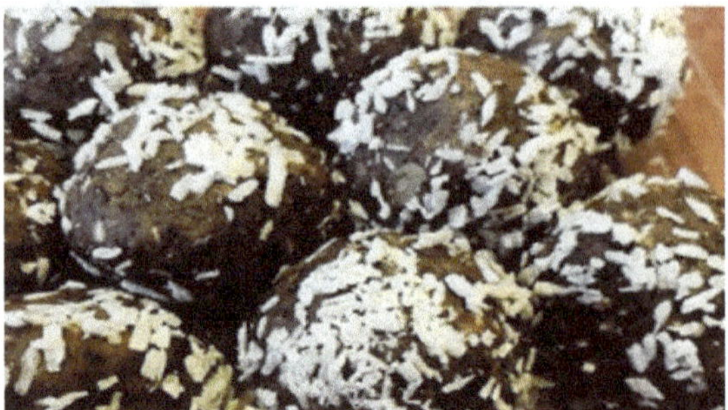

60g oats
120g tahini
4 tsp instant coffee or 2 tsp espresso coffee granules
2 tbs lactose free or almond milk
10g ground flaxseed
30g dark chocolate
1tbs maple syrup
2 tbs sesame seeds
Desiccated coconut to roll

Directions

1. Place oats in blender and process until flour-like consistecy
2. Transfer into a large bowl
3. Then place dark chocolate in food processor and blend until small pieces (or just use chips!)
4. Mix into oat flour
5. In small cup, stir together instant/espresso coffee and milk until coffee has dissolved
6. Add all the ingredients to the flour choc mix: coffee, tahini, ground flaxseeds, sesame seeds, maple syrup
7. Stir to combine well. If mixture is too dry, add more milk, 1 tsp at a time
8. Scoop out a tablespoon of mixture at a time and roll into balls using the palm of your hands.
9. Roll in coconut and pop into fridge until ready to eat!
10. Should keep in fridge for 2 weeks in an airtight container.

Loaded Veggie Nachos

Serves 2-4

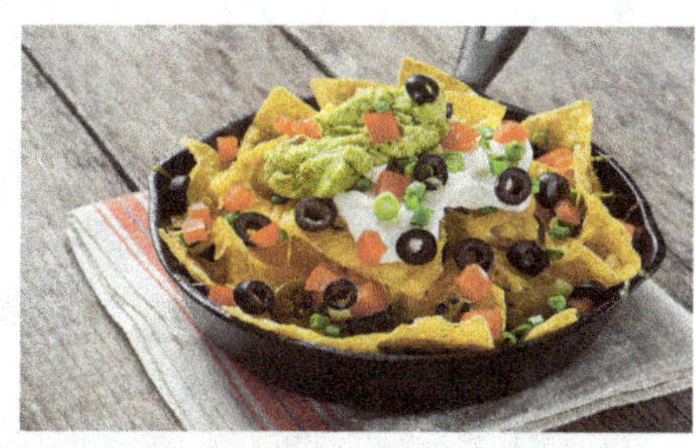

Ingredients

1 bag corn tortillas (ensure no onion or garlic in ingredients list)
120g cheddar cheese, grated
80g black beans, drained and rinsed
60g black olives, sliced
1 medium tomato, diced
Jarred roasted red pepper, diced
1/2 small avocado
2 scallions, green parts only, diced
100g lactose free yoghurt or low fat creme fraiche, if desired

Directions

1. Preheat the oven to 160 degrees and line a baking sheet with foil.
2. Place a single layer of chips on your baking sheet and sprinkle with half of the cheese and black beans
3. Make a second layer of chips and sprinkle the remaining cheese and black beans.
4. Bake for 5 minutes (or until cheese has melted).
5. Mash the avocado with diced tomato and sprinkle with black pepper
6. Remove nachos and top with avo-tomato mix, scallions, black olives and red pepper
7. Place dollops of yoghurt on top.
8. Serve immediately

MISCELLANEOUS

Making your FODMAP Life easy!

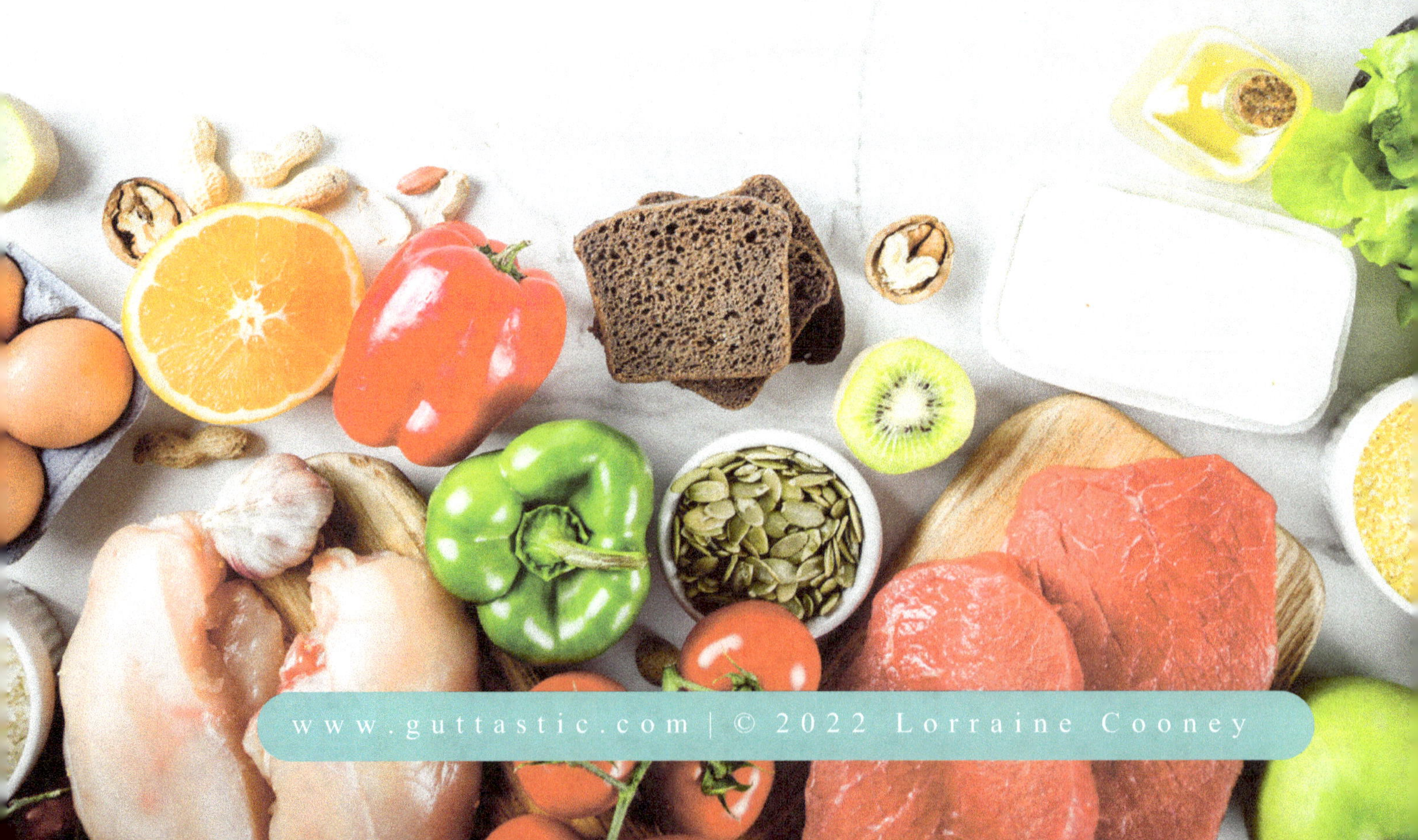

Easy Chicken Stock

Serves 4L

Ingredients

1 tsp garlic infused oil
1 chicken/or leftover cooked chicken, cut up into 6-8 pieces
2 carrots, cut into chunks
2 celery stalks, cut into chunks
1 turnip, cut into chunks
Handful of fresh herbs (e.g. parsley, thyme and rosemary)
Handful of fresh chives, finely chopped
3 bay leaves
1 tsp whole peppercorns
1L cold water
Salt and pepper to season

Directions

1. Heat the oil in a large saucepan
2. Place all the ingredients into the saucepan and cover with cold water (about 3L) and season
3. Bring to the boil, reduce the heat and simmer for 1.5 to 2 hours.
4. As it cooks, skim any impurities on the surface.
5. When done, pull any meat left on the chicken for another use (e.g. salads, sandwiches)
6. Strain the broth and discard all the non-liquid leftovers
7. Can freeze in portions for use later

Veg Boullion Stock Cubes

Serves 40

Ingredients

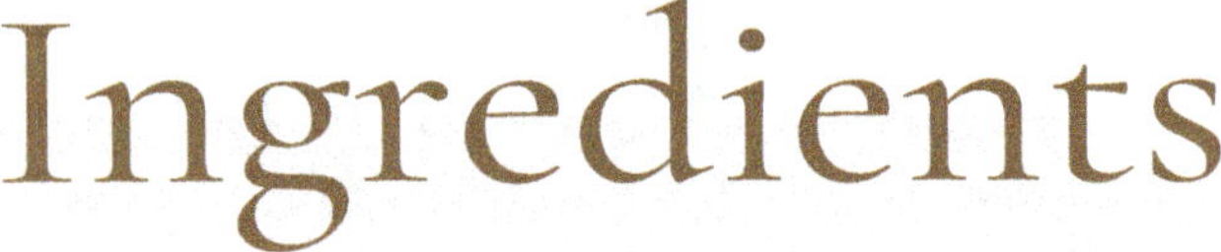

1 medium carrot, chopped into chunky pieces
5 sun-dried tomatoes
4 spring onions (green part only)
1/2 green pepper, roughly chopped
2 radishes, halved
1 tbs chives
Handful of fresh coriander
Handful of fresh parsley
1 tsp white pepper
1 tsp salt

Directions

1.Place the carrot, sun-dried tomatoes, spring onion, green pepper and radish in a food processor and blend until all ingredients are finely chopped
2.The add the fresh herbs, pepper and salt
3.Blend together until you have a smooth paste
4.This can be used immediately (approx.1tsp/600ml water)
5.Put the remainder into ice cube trays and freeze
6.Remove when frozen and store individually ice-cubes in a zip lock bag for when needed

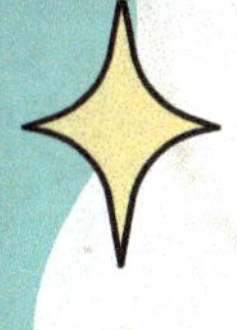

MY DAILY
notes

Date :

M T W T F

notes :

today's focus :

goals :

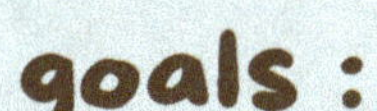

priorities :

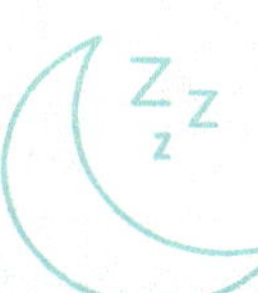

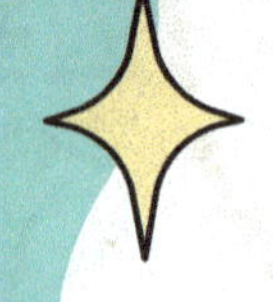

MY DAILY
notes

Date :

M T W T F

notes :

today's focus :

goals :

priorities :

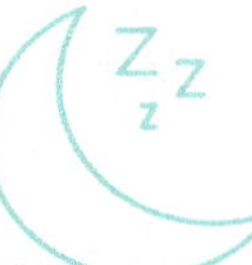

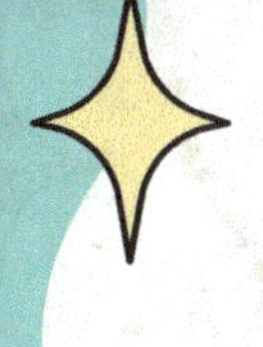

MY DAILY
notes

Date :

M T W T F

notes :

today's focus :

goals :

priorities :

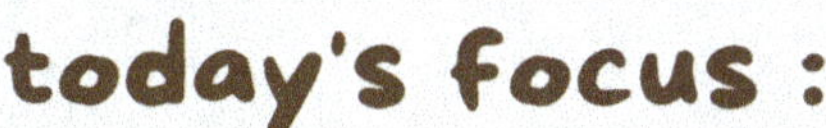

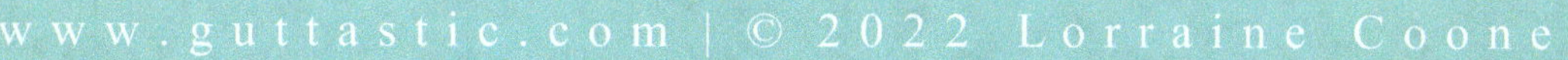

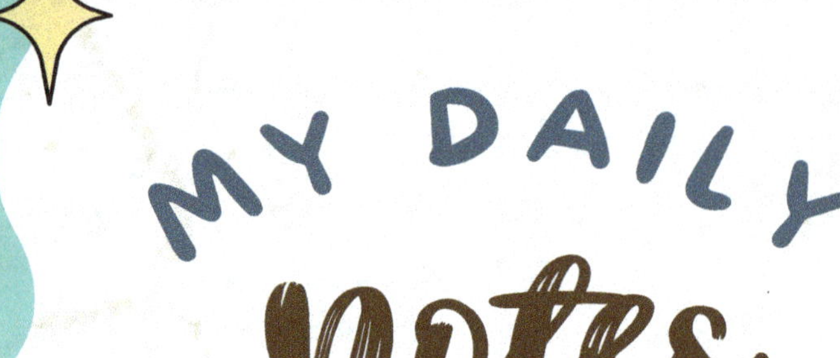

MY DAILY
notes

Date :

M T W T F

notes :

today's focus :

goals :

priorities :

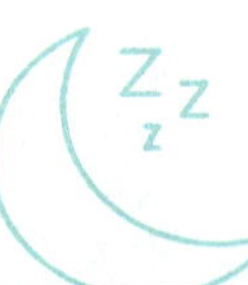

MY DAILY
notes

Date :

M T W T F

notes :

today's focus :

goals :

priorities :

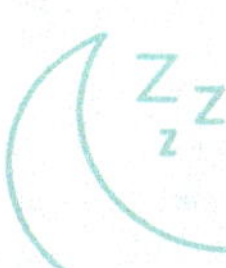

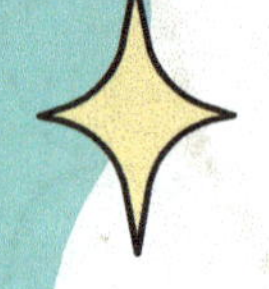

MY DAILY
notes

Date :

M T W T F

notes :

today's focus :

goals :

priorities :

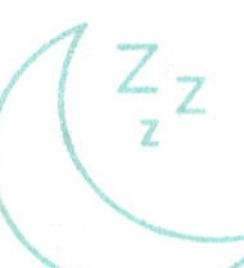

GROCERY LIST

VEGETABLES & FRUITS

GRAINS

DAIRY/NON-DAIRY

PROTEIN

NUTS. SEEDS. PULSES

CONDIMENTS

OTHERS

GROCERY LIST

VEGETABLES & FRUITS

GRAINS

DAIRY/NON-DAIRY

PROTEIN

NUTS, SEEDS, PULSES

CONDIMENTS

OTHERS

GROCERY LIST

VEGETABLES & FRUITS

GRAINS

DAIRY/NON-DAIRY

PROTEIN

NUTS, SEEDS, PULSES

CONDIMENTS

OTHERS

GROCERY LIST

VEGETABLES & FRUITS

GRAINS

DAIRY/NON-DAIRY

PROTEIN

NUTS. SEEDS. PULSES

CONDIMENTS

OTHERS

GROCERY LIST

VEGETABLES & FRUITS

GRAINS

DAIRY/NON-DAIRY

PROTEIN

NUTS, SEEDS, PULSES

CONDIMENTS

OTHERS

GROCERY LIST

VEGETABLES & FRUITS

GRAINS

DAIRY/NON-DAIRY

PROTEIN

NUTS. SEEDS. PULSES

CONDIMENTS

OTHERS

MEAL PLANNER

WEEK OF: _____________

	BREAKFAST	LUNCH	DINNER	SNACKS
MON				
TUE				
WED				
THU				
FRI				
SAT				
SUN				

MEAL PLANNER

WEEK OF: _______________

	BREAKFAST	LUNCH	DINNER	SNACKS
MON				
TUE				
WED				
THU				
FRI				
SAT				
SUN				

MEAL PLANNER

WEEK OF: _______________

	BREAKFAST	LUNCH	DINNER	SNACKS
MON				
TUE				
WED				
THU				
FRI				
SAT				
SUN				

MEAL PLANNER

WEEK OF: _______________

	BREAKFAST	LUNCH	DINNER	SNACKS
MON				
TUE				
WED				
THU				
FRI				
SAT				
SUN				

MEAL PLANNER

WEEK OF: _____________

	BREAKFAST	LUNCH	DINNER	SNACKS
MON				
TUE				
WED				
THU				
FRI				
SAT				
SUN				

MEAL PLANNER

WEEK OF: ___________

	BREAKFAST	LUNCH	DINNER	SNACKS
MON				
TUE				
WED				
THU				
FRI				
SAT				
SUN				

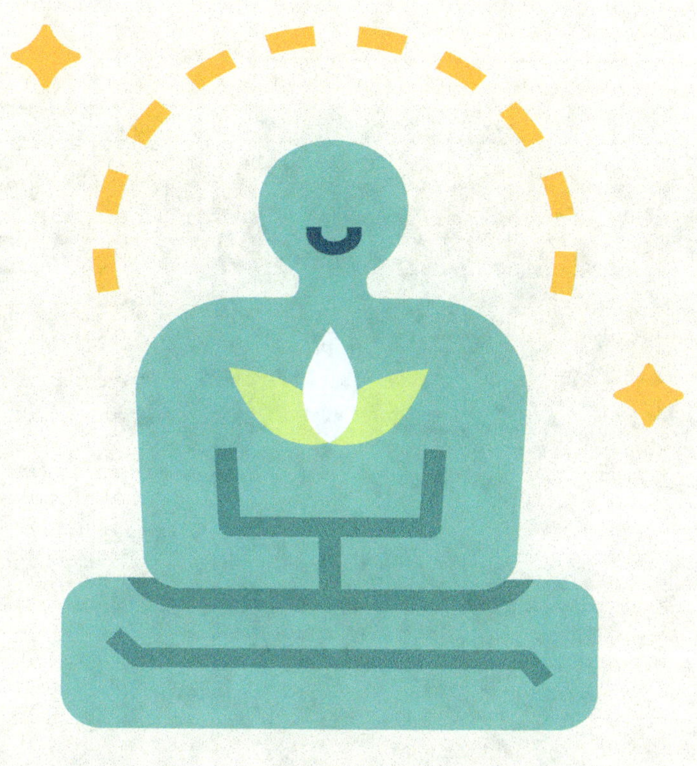

HAVE QUESTIONS?

Please email: info@guttastic.com

"WITH YOUR GUT, EVERY DAY IS A LEARNING DAY!"

LORRAINE COONEY